I0437347

THE CURTAIN
NEVER MOVED

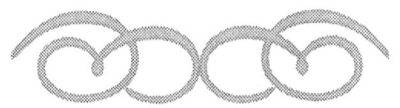

Jess Barker

Bloomington, IN 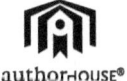 Milton Keynes, UK

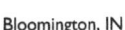

authorHOUSE®

AuthorHouse™
1663 Liberty Drive, Suite 200
Bloomington, IN 47403
www.authorhouse.com
Phone: 1-800-839-8640

AuthorHouse™ UK Ltd.
500 Avebury Boulevard
Central Milton Keynes, MK9 2BE
www.authorhouse.co.uk
Phone: 08001974150

© 2006 Jess Barker. All rights reserved.

*No part of this book may be reproduced, stored in
a retrieval system, or transmitted by any means
without the written permission of the author.*

First published by AuthorHouse 11/30/2006

ISBN: 978-1-4259-6868-7 (sc)

Printed in the United States of America
Bloomington, Indiana

This book is printed on acid-free paper.

Introduction

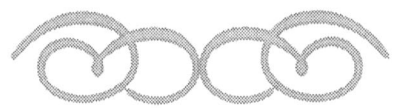

*T*his story I write is not intended to cause hurt to any of my dear brothers or sisters, or to disturb the memories they choose to try and forget, so they can block out the violence, the mental abuse, the loneliness and the anger that disturbed all of our lives, this enables them to lead a normal life.

Understanding this I have to protect my brothers, sisters and other family members, therefore I respect their wishes as I tell my story and not name them by their real names.

The story I tell is a true account from start to end of how my life as a child, which started with happiness and love was then suddenly turned upside down into a tormented world of abuse, violence and survival. How from a timid child I became a strong minded woman who soon understood that this period of my life was not normal.

Yet people of authority ignored my many pleas for help and even made matters worse by making me feel more insecure, rejected and alone.

Despite the cruel life I endured as a child I thankfully grew up wanting my own children to have the love, security, respect and family life that I had so yearned for. In truth I wanted to keep the love mum gave me alive.

Dedication

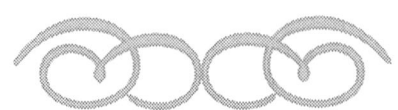

I would like to say a special thank you to my beloved family who have helped and supported me and have had the patience and understanding of my emotions of frustration and anger as I have relived this time in my life which has enabled me to tell my story.

I would also like to say a special thank you to a special friend Martin James House. He gave me the strength, support and courage I needed and helped me to understand and believe in myself. He gave me the security I never had and kept me alive when I was so alone.

Also thank you Martin for helping me Find the appropriate Title for my book.

Chapter 1

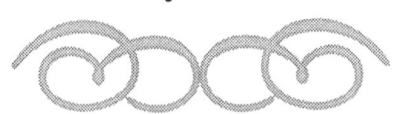

WARMTH OF A MOTHERS LOVE

Remembering back to when I was four years of age. Mum was a bubbly lady, always had a smile, always busy but never too busy to give us a hug and kiss us and tell us how much she loved us. She always kept the house clean, was always cooking and kept me and my brothers and sisters looking nice.

Mum was called Rose and she had black wavy shoulder length hair, and always wore an apron that I recall, she was always cheerful with a twinkle in her eyes. Mum was proud of all of her children. My eldest sister Jane lived at home, my second eldest sister Sandy was married to Allen who was tall, dark and handsome man they had a son of their own also called Allen but they lived in the same street as us, my third eldest sister Lizzie lived at home along with my three older brothers Jake, Paul and Roy.

Many people would say I was mums double in looks her high cheek bones her smile. We were all happy living in a secure environment which centred around mum, mum did her best to provide and we never went short of love and affection or food.

I shared a double bed with my two older sisters in the upstairs front bedroom of our house in Cellars road, in the city of London.

Mum was a popular lady and got on with everyone, we had two cats, Ben and Sleepy, mum adored them and Ben was Lizzie's cat. I never knew mum to go out, in the summer she would go and visit her parents in Essex where her Father worked on a farm on her return she would have bags full of onions, green beans, carrots and other vegetables all fresh from the farm.

Our Father, well he was always in and out, he was the opposite of mum, stern and too strict, as young as I was I remember getting a beating for standing on an empty bird cage. I cannot recall one time he ever showed us any love or affection. Mum tried to protect us as much as she could. Our Father had aviaries in the back garden with Budgies, Canaries and Finches. We had a goat, ducks and chickens as well as the two cats. It was little house on the prairie the animals were his pride and joy.

With mum we were happy we were her pride and joy. Soon I was to start school and I remember mum telling me how good it was at school how she would take me with the others and get me at home time. Christmases were a time to remember too, we always had a stocking full of goodies and the Christmas when I was five, me and Lizzie were given a silver cross pram which was our pride and joy, later on my brothers stole the wheels from it to make a go cart.

I had no worries to think about mum made home happy and secure. Our Father, Ed was a different story the only affection he showed us was his belt and a kiss goodnight which was through routine not choice. The time passed and things seemed to change, being too young to understand I plodded along. Mum went away on a few occasions, I thought she had gone to the farm but later on I found out from my older sisters that this was when Mum went to hospital. I do remember walking to the hospital in London as a family and waving to mum through the window and blowing her kisses while she blew kisses to all of us. I didn't understand what was going on because in those days no one talked in front of the children, children were seen and not heard.

I remember my two older sisters Jane and Sandy saying mum wasn't well and we had to be extra good. Mum and Dad had the front room downstairs as their bedroom, the boys had the middle and back rooms upstairs.

We had no bathroom, bath days meant the old tin bath had to be dragged in from the garden and set up in front of the open fire and then it was one in one out, or we would be sent over to the family across the road where Mrs B, Mums friend would bath us, this happened more when mum was ill.

At the time when mum was ill our Father seemed very uptight and extra snappy and moody, more so than usual. Suddenly people were in and out of house more so now, than ever before.

Sandy would come around to take us to school.

We came home one day and mum was not there, we were told that she was in hospital and that she would be home soon and that was all we were told. We were allowed to go and play outside in the street as we often did. As me and Roy were sitting on the pavement a Lady approached us and asked us if we were Ed's kids! Roy nudged me with his elbow and asked me who she was because he had seen her outside the house before but I didn't know her. As we hadn't answered her the first time she asked us again rather sternly if we were Ed's kids, we both looked up and said "Yes". She then asked us if our Father was at home but he wasn't so she turned and walked back up the street.

Roy then told me that she had been at the house before asking for Dad and when he went inside to tell him there was a woman outside asking for him, Dad had taken one look at the woman and turned to Roy and smacked him round the head and sent him up to bed. Roy didn't understand what he had done wrong, he had only passed on a message so from that day on Roy didn't like that woman. When he told me I just said "Dad did that because he's nutty, but Lizzie was frightened to hear me talking about Dad like that and told me not to say things like that because I would get in trouble but I didn't care I laughed and said "but he is".

Well the days went by, soon mum was home and spent her days in bed, we were only allowed to enter her room with an adult, which we did once in the morning and once at night. Mum was always pleased to see us, as we were her. Every time we saw her she would kiss and hug us and tell us how much she loved us.

It was the end of September and I remember making her a birthday card, when I gave it to her she held it close to her and a tear ran down her cheek, "that's lovely" she said and hugged me and planted kisses all over my face. She held my hand and said "never forget that I love you", she then reminded me that it would be my birthday soon and that I would be a big seven, I had to promise her that I would a good girl which she made us do whenever we saw her. I promised her I would and told her that I loved her too, she cried when I said that and then I had to leave the room as she was getting tired.

It was about this time that our two older sisters, Jane and Sandy seemed to be doing more for us, like washing us, helping us get ready for school and generally care for us and love us as mum had done before she had become ill. I remember saying to Sandy that she was being like mummy, she hugged and kissed me when I said that but I noticed a sadness in her eyes as she told me to run along.

Our Father had a busy life doing allsorts. One of his hobbies before mum was ill was doing magic, he held the world record for being buried alive for so many minutes, in the early 60's he did flame throwing and would lay on a bed of nails. He called himself Great Kara. For a living he was a cabinet maker or a wood machinist as he called himself.

Mum was the homemaker but when she was ill things changed that even became noticeable to us younger ones too, no one was allowed to ask questions we were all just told to run along and play.

Our street was a blocked turning, round the corner was where my eldest sister lived with her family, she came to see us everyday. Sandy, Jane and Mum would chat for hours, Sandy's baby son Allen was mums first grandchild and she adored him and spoilt him. I remember her saying that when she was better she would take Allen out for the day. She would tell me I was his auntie but I didn't understand that as I thought you had to be a grownup to be an auntie, I thought mum was joking I would say how can I be an auntie I'm not even seven yet. She tried to explain but it was all too confusing, to me he was a baby, Sandy's baby and that was that. I was more interested in where the baby came from but no one wanted to tell me that.

Mum was a very caring person, a few years earlier Paul was playing on a rope that was bound round a street light taking turns to swing with Jake. I'm not sure what happened but Paul somehow fell forward and smashed his face on the lamp post, biting into his tongue. Mum was there to calm him, cuddle him and to reassure him, Paul was taken inside, as upset as Paul was mum never left his side.

On another occasion Paul was ill, doubled in pain, I remember mum calling for an ambulance. Paul was carried out over the ambulance mans shoulder into the ambulance, mum never left his side, she was very upset her son was ill and the concern showed in her face and actions, as she was there to love and reassure him again. It turns out he had appendicitis and had to have his appendix removed. Mum was unsettled until her son returned home so she could care for him and nurse him better, those magic kisses always worked and before long he was boasting and showing us his scar.

Our Jake spent most of his school holidays and weekend's at work with Dad. Jake never wanted to go he would have preferred to stay with Mum. But Jake had no choice as far as Dad was concerned. I believe Jake resented not being allowed to stay at home with mum.

Going back not so long before mum was ill I remember going out with her to a big building as we entered she told me to be quiet because we were playing a game. We went into a big room which echoed with tables and gadgets, no one was around then we heard voices and giggling. Mum told me to hide under the table and put her finger to her lips sshhhh! We didn't make a sound. The voices echoed around the room and I recognised Dads voice as I looked to see where the voices were coming from I saw Dad with a woman in his arms, mum pulled me back still with her finger to her lips, I looked at her and watched the tears roll down her face. Soon Dad and the woman went, we had to wait until it went quiet before we emerged from our hiding place as we went outside mum turned to me, smiled wiped her eyes and said "come along let's go home". She told me we had just been playing hide and seek and not to tell Dad. Mum seemed very quiet on the way home and kept hugging me and touching my face. We had tea not long after we got in and then went to bed before Dad got home as she tucked me in and gave me a goodnight kiss she put her finger to her lips and said sshhhh! again.

That night we heard shouting, Dads voice over Mums and then the door slammed as Dad went out we then heard the van engine start.

Dad was the only one in our street with a van. On one occasion I remember Lizzie sitting on the step of the van swinging her legs without a care in the world, next thing she was being dragged indoors with Dad shouting at her and hitting her. She ran away from him and went and hid behind mum, Dad told Mum to give Lizzie to him but Mum told Lizzie to run and hide. Mum then began shouting at Dad, not to hit Lizzie, Dad then stormed out. Mum then asked Lizzie what she had done to make Dad hit her like that but Lizzie said that she didn't know. We realised it was just because she was sitting on the step of the Van but we couldn't see what harm she could have been doing just sitting there but no one dared to say anything for fear of getting the same. In the mornings as Dad went out to work mum stood at the gate with us waiting until he got to the end of the turning, he would stop at the greengrocers and come out with an orange and roll it down the hill towards mum so she would fetch it and cut it up for us all to have a piece. Once we were washed and dressed mum went out and about and fed the cats and other animals. I can never remember mum just sitting down she was always on the go. The mats went on the line and she would beat them clean with a broom. She would then go on her hands and knees and scrub the floors, always busy keeping the home and us nice.

On one occasion I remember mum putting a little make up on after she had washed her face and had got tea ready, she did this so that she looked nice for Dad when he got in. She would put her lipstick on and then dab it dry with one of Dads handkerchiefs and this particular day he came home and saw her with her lipstick on and demanded to see his handkerchief when he saw the lipstick marks on it he shouted at her and then demanded his tea. I could see this had really upset her she called me to her, placed a tea towel over my hands, placed his hot dinner on the tea towel and told me to take it to my Father. He was still shouting at mum at this point and as I walked towards him he got louder and louder demanding I hurry up with his dinner as I got in front of him I threw his dinner in the air and it went over his head and down his front into his lap. I ran as fast as I could back into the scullery to hide behind mum, as I peeped round her legs I could see the anger on his face. As he stood the food dropped off him onto the floor and as he headed towards us mum pushed me further behind her while pleading with him that I didn't mean to do it but it was no good, as Dad got to mum he reached behind her and grabbed me by the arm and started hitting me across my legs, arms, back and face. Mum pulled me back towards her and he stormed out.

Mum began cuddling me and rubbing the red marks he had left she told me I was a silly girl and I mustn't do that, through the sobs I said "but he upset you again and I don't like him" she said "you mustn't say that about your Father". She quickly got me washed and dressed and into bed before he came home.

Jane went to help clear up the food on the chair and floor and as she spoke to mum I saw a smile on mums face and then I was glad I had done it.

As I mentioned Dad kept lots of animals and at one time helped out at a the local zoo and would sometimes bring sick animal's home to nurture them back to health but as the animals would find out his idea of nurturing was not as yours or mine.

On one occasion he brought home a chimpanzee which I thought was really cute, but he was soon to be mentally and physically abused just like the rest of us. Dad would torment the chimp with a banana and lock it in a long dark wooden box and the chimp would screech and bang the sides of the box. When he finally let it out it would go mad, biting and pulling at anyone in its way. We all felt sorry for it and while Dad was out mum would let him out of the box and cuddle him like a baby and the chimp would lay in mums arms calm and enjoying the affection. Mum was just so caring to everyone and everything.

People were always in and out of our house, Aunts, Uncles, Cousins and Neighbours, the doors were always left open back then, you could go out and come back to nothing touched. My Brother

Roy and I used to sit on the door step with a chunk of bread and dripping and watch people go by, because Roy had eaten his lunch mum gave him one sweet, but for some reason dad objected to this and belted Roy and sent him to bed where he had to stay for six weeks, only being allowed down to eat dinner of a night and had to be back in bed before dad got in, no one question dad's ruling although mum did as she thought this was a bit too harsh as Roy hadn't done nothing wrong, but the ruling had to stay, no one was allowed to go up and play or talk to him. But mum did, she was up and down all day to see him.

The Neighbours next door on the left loved Roy and a few times they asked mum if they could adopt him, "oh no" my mum would say. They would always buy him sweets and rub the top of his head, they had no children of their own and they loved our Roy. Mum would share the sweets they bought him out between us all. Roy would say smiling "that lady said I was special" mum would reply "you are all special my love".

Sundays we were all dressed in our best clothes, I used to think we were going out but was told by mum that we just had to wear our Sunday best clothes I never understood why and gave up asking in the end. Every Friday mum would give us   2d and we were allowed to go to the top of the road to the sweet shop in Winter Lane next to the off licence. It was 1/2d for three mojo chews or blackjacks, we would come back and sit on the pavement and eat them, happy as Larry not a care in the world.

By now mum had taken to her bed and I didn't understand why, I was too young to figure it out and when I asked no one would give me an answer.

Chapter 2

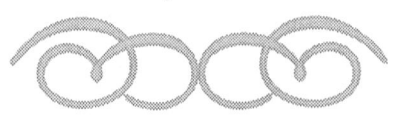

No Goodbyes

Soon it was a mild morning in October, I overheard our Jane say October already, I jumped up and shouted "yes" then mum said it would be my birthday soon but to keep the noise down and put the cat, sleepy out. As I did this I turned to Jane and asked her what happened to sleep's kittens that she had given birth to a few months before, I wanted to know what had happened to the one that had been sat on and squashed by a lady that had come round to see mum, I remember mum being very upset and trying to make the kitten better but couldn't remember what happened after that. Jane told me it had gone up to heaven then she said I had to hurry up and get to school. I didn't want to go to school that day, I wanted to stay home but I was not allowed so I went in to see mum and gave her a hug and kiss as usual like the others all did. She was sat up in her bed, as she was expecting us, she had a big smile on her face, she told us all to be good and that she would see us all that night I noticed she was holding her hand over her tummy.

Over the next few days Mum seemed tired all the time and pale, none of us knew why she remained in bed or what was wrong, we kids weren't told anything. We got home from school one night and it had got dark early, I had drawn mum a picture I wanted to give it to her as soon as we got in but tea was nearly ready and we were told to play for a while, after tea we had to get washed and dressed for bed and only then were we allowed to see mum. We all went in together, Jane, Sandy, Jake, Paul, Lizzie, Roy, me. She was propped up in bed with a smile on her face. I gave her the picture I had been anxious to give her all night, as she took it tears rolled down her face, she told me it was lovely as she took my hand in hers and kissed it she reminded me that it would be my seventh birthday within days. We all sat around her and took it in turns to tell her the events of our day; she told us all to be good children and told us how much she loved us all. I didn't think anything strange at that she was always telling us how much she loved us and how much we were all special to her. But that night we had to pray together that was very strange because we had never had to say prayers before but we all said prayers and no one questioned why. Soon we were told it was bedtime and that mum needed to rest, as we got up we took it in turns to give mum kisses and cuddles and she reminded us all to be good for mummy. With all the goodnights said we went off to bed.

The next morning I was awoken by a muffled strange sound I wasn't sure what it was but I knew it didn't sound right. I began to feel frightened, I got out of bed and walked towards the door, I hesitated opening the door I held the door knob pulling it back slowly, the wider the door opened the louder the sound became, my heart was racing. By now the door was wide open but there was no one on the landing, the noise seemed to echo in the hallway. I knew something was terribly wrong, my stomach was churning and I felt sick. I slowly walked towards the stairs I stepped down a few steps onto the top of the stairs, I wasn't sure what it was I was hearing whether it was real or if it was just another one of my nightmares that seemed so real at times. I put my hand over my face and spread my fingers wide and peeped through the gaps which was something I did when I was really scared. It was real, as there at the bottom of the stairs were my brothers and sisters sobbing with their faces in their hands unable to control their emotions. I looked over the banister and saw our Father stood between mums room and the spare room facing the front door. I began to slowly walk down the stairs; my knees were shaking, what could be so wrong I thought. I removed my hand from my face and stopped halfway down the stairs, I seemed to have frozen in fear, and I felt sick. Jane saw me standing there and held out her hand for me to grasp, her face was red and swollen and her eyes were blood shot, her outstretched hand was shaking, I took it hesitantly and walked the rest of the way down the stairs. At this point I realised it was something to do with mum and I started to cry and shake. Jane pulled me towards her and tucked me into her stomach and put her arm around me tightly to protect me. We all tried to quieten down by putting our hands over our mouths to try and muffle our sobbing noise, I realised now that this was the sound that had awoken me. Jane had one hand over her mouth and one hand wrapped around me. Then mums bedroom door opened and we saw a tall grey haired man dressed in black walking backwards out of the room and talking in a stern voice to someone inside the room, for some reason I knew he wasn't talking to mum. As he stepped back he had his arms in front and was holding a stretcher which he was turning towards the front door, the stretcher was covered in a white sheet and there was another tall man holding the other end. I just knew that it was mum under that sheet and I shouted at the men to leave her alone, I tried to escape Jane's grip to rescue mum but she held me tight with both her hands on my shoulders. "NO"! She said holding me with a tight grip. Sandy was holding Roy on one side of her and Paul and Jake the other, she was trying to comfort them and control her own emotions at the same time. Sandy turned towards the kitchen area taking the boys with her, Jane and I followed, all of us sobbing uncontrollably. Our Father shut the front door as the men went out. In the kitchen area we found Lizzie hiding behind the folding doors, she had been too scared to come out. As young as I was I just for some strange reason knew we weren't going to see mum again, I didn't really understand what was happening. We were sat down and calmed down; we were passed a cup of sweet tea and were told to drink it down. I wanted to ask where they had taken our mum but I was scared to ask as I was afraid of the answer. After we drank our tea Sandy and Jane took us up to get dressed, they told us we had to be good children and kept kissing and hugging us as mum did.

We were made to eat a little breakfast and taken to school by Sandy and her husband Allen when we got there they chatted to our teachers very quietly.

I still did not quite understand what had actually happened that morning but I was feeling scared and uptight but the day was kept as normal. After school we were taken home which was full of people talking softly, next we were taken away from home and Lizzie and I went with Aunt Sadie I don't remember to this day how we got to her house. We arrived and we were shown where we would be sleeping. Aunt Sadie took me upstairs to a room that had a double bed in it that had a cot beside it I was told that it was hers and Uncle

Geoff's room and that I would be sleeping in the cot. I looked at her and told her that I didn't sleep in a cot anymore but she just replied that while I was staying there I would have to sleep in it. We went back downstairs to the kitchen area where Lizzie was waiting; I went and sat next to her. All I kept thinking about was the night before with us all huddled around mum saying prayers and listening as she told us all to be good and reminded us how much she loved us all while kissing and cuddling each of us in turn. Thinking now I did notice that her expressions were different as she spoke to us that night but I had just thought it was because she was tired and it was past our bedtime. As I was recalling the events of last night I was soon snapped back to reality by Aunt Sadie's voice telling me that my tea was ready, as I headed to the table she remarked "you were in a world of your own then dear, you had best snap out of it and look lively". After tea Aunt Sadie cleared away the dishes as I went and sat next to Lizzie, I felt safer being with her, it didn't feel right being at Aunt Sadie's house I wanted to go home. I thought back to that morning when Sandy and Jane were getting us dressed and them telling us to be good and that they loved us as we sobbed we had nodded in agreement. Next thing I knew Aunt Sadie's face was close to mine she said "you were in a world of your own again, come on girl up to bed a good nights sleep will do you good." I was lead upstairs through a door in the kitchen, it was cold and dark and all the time I was wishing I could go home. Aunt Sadie told me I was on a little holiday that was why I was staying with her, she then helped me into the cot, I didn't want to go in the cot I didn't understand why I had to go in there as I wasn't a baby. When Aunt Sadie left I was alone in the dark with only the street light shining in I was very scared and confused and cried myself to sleep. The next morning I awoke needing to go to the toilet as I turned over the cot creaked and woke up Uncle Geoff, he yawned and asked me what time it was, I said I didn't know and that I needed to go to the toilet. He woke up Aunt Sadie who took me downstairs and out the back where the toilet was or carsey as they called it. Aunt Sadie said to me "hurry up girl its cold out here", as we came back in she ordered me to sit on the chair and not to wake Lizzie up yet as she was asleep on a bed behind the sofa. Aunt Sadie put the kettle on and then went back upstairs leaving me shivering on the chair. Uncle Geoff and Aunt

Sadie came back down and I was told to go up and get dressed and not to take too long, when I came back down Lizzie was awake, she half smiled at me as she got up, I could see that she had been crying as her face was all swollen. My thoughts returned to yesterday morning and then tears started to roll down my face again. I wondered if it had been a nightmare and I wanted to ask Lizzie about it but I was scared to in case Aunt Sadie overheard me. Aunt Sadie asked us if we liked porridge we both said that we did and then were told to sit up the table. When I got my porridge I took a mouthful and straight away spat it out saying "yuk that tastes salty". Aunt Sadie said "oh god child just eat up" "I can't" I said "it's horrible" "well go and sit over there and go without" she said and told me to drink my tea, as she warned me not to spill it. Nervously I drank my tea.

I didn't like it here much, I started to cry again, "what are you snivelling now for child" Aunt Sadie said "I want to go home and see my mum" I replied. "Well child you can't go home yet" she said in a stern voice. I wondered what she meant by that but I was too scared to ask her, I was told to be quiet and to drink my tea. I hated it here already I thought, Lizzie was always quiet and never spoke to anyone, she did what she was told and asked no questions, she was a shy person at the best of times. We spent most of that day just sitting around as there was nothing much to do, there was a telly in the corner above Uncle Geoff's' chair but it only went on at night time and even then we weren't allowed to watch it. Soon it was dark outside and Uncle Geoff came in, he took his overcoat off along with his cap and boots and slumped himself in his chair and that is where he stayed most of the night. He looked at us and said in his deep voice "have you two behaved yourselves today?" we both just nodded yes. He then told us to go and get changed for bed, neither of us said a word we were too scared to and he frightened us. "Well" Uncle Geoff asked again. "Lost your tongues girls" he snapped.

We didn't say a word, just got up and went upstairs. Uncle Geoff and Aunt Sadie were talking and stopped as we entered back into the room but I had managed to hear the word funeral. I thought to myself that I had heard that word before and thought back to the day when a little girl was killed by a van in our street outside our house, a few days later a big black car had come down our street "for her funeral" someone had told me but

I didn't know what it meant but I was scared that Aunt Sadie and Uncle Geoff were talking about a funeral. Next thing I knew I was being told to look lively by Aunt Sadie as tea was ready as I sat up the table I was handed a plate type bowl full of stew Aunt Sadie told me to stop day dreaming and to eat up because we had a busy day tomorrow so we had to hurry up and eat so that we could go to bed. I started crying again "what you snivelling for now girl" Aunt Sadie said I told her I wanted to go home and see my mum and asked her where my Jane, Sandy, Paul, Roy, Jake were. She didn't answer me and just rubbed my head and asked if I would like to sleep in with Lizzie tonight? I just nodded yes; Lizzie put her arms around me and told me not to cry as she was there for me. Lizzie was not much older than me; she was coming up to eleven. After a while we climbed into bed and collapsed with the exhaustion of all the crying we had been doing. We lay in each others arms and cried ourselves to sleep. Next morning I was awoken by Uncle Geoff lighting the fire and Aunt Sadie clunking cups on the table. Uncle Geoff said "morning" as he yawned I said "morning" in return he said that breakfast was ready so to wake Lizzie, I gently shook her awake. We ate breakfast and then went and got washed and dressed. Aunt Sadie had our old case packed by the door, as I spotted it I asked her if this meant we were going home today she replied "no not today" I asked her why our case was there then she said in a soft voice "you'll see why soon" Lizzie and I just looked at each other "the 13th today isn't it Sadie?" Uncle Geoff asked "yes and unlucky for some at that" She replied. With that Uncle Geoff put on his overcoat, his boots and his cap and said "cheerio and behave yourselves girls" and off he went out the front door. Aunt Sadie put our night clothes into the case by the door and then came and sat down with a cup of tea she told us that we going to go and stay with Uncle Ollie and Aunt Val, just for a few days and that Aunt Val would be arriving soon to pick us up, as she rose to her feet again, Lizzie and I just held each others hands and sat in silence. Aunt Sadie went about tidying up and there was soon a bang at the door, Aunt Sadie opened it up and Aunt Val came through saying good morning to Aunt Sadie and then to Lizzie and I. Soon we were on our way to Aunt Val and Uncle Ollie's house.

Chapter 3

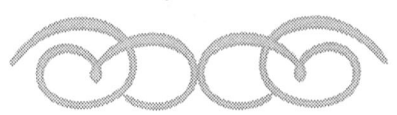

PILLAR TO POST

*N*ow we were more confused than ever and felt very afraid as we did not know what was happening, all we knew was that we were being sent to stay with another relative. On our journey to Aunt Val's house she told us that we would be staying with her as a little holiday and that we would be attending a different school for awhile. Lizzie and I asked her where our Brothers and Sisters were, but as Aunt Sadie had done before she changed the subject quickly so as to avoid answering us. As we arrived at her house she said "come on in girls, lets pop your case in and then we can go and see your new school." I held Lizzie's hand tight and began to cry. "I've got my own school" I sobbed "It's only for a little while dear" Aunt Val said with a smile. We walked for a while, I never let go of Lizzie's hand no one said a word and tears just rolled down my face. "Here we are girls" Aunt Val said as we approached the school in Moore's Lane. We walked through the main doors and a woman approached us. "You must be the Barker girls" she said.

She did introduce herself to us but I wasn't listening, I just wanted to go home, I didn't want to be there at all. After she chatted with Aunt Val we were lead off by the lady and taken to a classroom. She left me on a chair and turned and took Lizzie off to another classroom. I was still crying and all the children were staring at me and whispering to each other which made me cry even more. "Oh dear" said the teacher "you poor mite, let me sort something out" next I was being lead out of the classroom by the teacher and into the one that Lizzie had been sent to. "There you might be better left with your sister for today" the teacher said and left to go back to her own classroom. I sat with Lizzie and straight away felt a bit better. I noticed that she was shaking head to toe as well. "Why are we here?" I asked Lizzie "because the school," replied Lizzie "but I don't like it here, I want to go home and go to my own school" I said. "Well you can't" said Lizzie "Why not?" I cried "We just can't that's why" Lizzie said sternly but I noticed that she was crying to, the school day eventually came to an end and we were shown to the front gate where Aunt Val was waiting, as she was asking if we had had a nice day the teacher called her over and they began talking quietly together. When we arrived back at Aunt Val's she told us to go in and make ourselves at home she said that she had put our case upstairs and that she would help us unpack it later. She put the tea on and then got some games out for us to play and while the tea was cooking she sat and played them with us. Just as tea was ready Uncle Ollie came in and said hello to us "How was school?" he asked when we didn't answer he looked at Aunt Val and I noticed her wink at him "You'll be ok" he said as he rubbed the top of my head. We all had tea together then we had to unpack our case and get washed and ready for bed. We went back downstairs and Uncle Ollie read us a story and then we had to go to bed. Once we were settled in bed Aunt Val brought us up a cup of cocoa and tucked us in. It was certainly a different house hold to Aunt Sadie's, as I lay in bed I thought of mum and soon cried my self to sleep. The next morning I was awoken by Aunt Val gently shaking me and saying "Good morning dear, time to get up, breakfast is ready, the fires on downstairs and I've made you a nice cup of tea." She then went and woke up Lizzie. When we got downstairs Uncle Ollie said "good morning" to us he said "it's a bit chilly out so wrap up warm" he then gave us a sixpence each I couldn't believe that I had sixpence all to myself I thanked him for it and he told me with a chuckle to spend it wisely. After breakfast we got washed and dressed and Aunt Val said "we were off to school again today," my face just dropped at the thought of it but Aunt Val just said "you'll be fine dear and tomorrow it's your birthday so you have that to look forward to, and if you're good we will pop to the shop so that you can spend your sixpence". Lizzie looked at me and smiled as I sat next to her she said "It's nice here isn't it" I smiled and said "yes but I still want to go home" she kissed my face and said "we will soon".

On went our hats and coats on and off we went to the shops and on to school. It wasn't that bad at school that day I stayed with Lizzie again and the other kids were friendly the day went quickly and soon we were on our way to the school gate to meet Aunt Val. We stopped at the shop and spent the rest of our money on sweets and then walked to Aunt Val's house. After tea we had a bath and got changed for bed, Uncle Ollie sat and told us a story again and then we went off to bed. When I woke up the next morning Aunt Val said "Happy Birthday dear you are not going to school today as your Dad is going to be visiting you after breakfast." I jumped out of bed and shouted excitedly "Yes! Mum's coming we're going home today" Aunt Val quickly replied "No you are not going home just yet, your Dad is just coming because it's your birthday." I wasn't excited anymore now that I knew we weren't going home, or for the fact dad was coming alone. Lizzie gave me a kiss and said "Happy Birthday you're seven today". I said "but I wanted to she mum" as I cried again, but after breakfast we got dressed Uncle Ollie got up and smiled at us.

He bent over and kissed us all and then left the house. Soon after Dad came and wished me a Happy Birthday and gave me a present I said "where's my mum" Aunt Val replied quickly "she can't make it today dear." As she looked at dad,

Dad didn't say a word or stay long and I remember crying because I wanted to go with him so that I could see mum. I was just told that I would be going home soon. The day passed by with Uncle Ollie in and out, soon it was dark and he read us a bedtime story. Over the next few days we often asked about our Brothers and Sisters but no one would tell us anything. A few days later the house seemed quiet and strange and that Uncle Ollie had stayed at home, both him and Aunt Val had got dressed into smart clothes and spent the morning talking together in whispers. We were taken to school and I noticed that Lizzie was very quiet that day, and that night I noticed that when Uncle Ollie read us our bedtime story it wasn't as good as it was on the other nights. The days seemed to go by and it seemed like we had been there forever when out of the blue one when we got up one Aunt Val said "You are going home today girls," Lizzie and I jumped up and down and cheered. It had been nice at Aunt Val and Uncle Ollie's house but I was missing home and missing my Mum and Brothers and Sisters. I couldn't eat my breakfast that morning and to this day I can't remember how we got home and who took us. I remember going through the front door to be meet by out

Nan, our faces dropped "where's my mum?" I asked Nan "slow down" she said "your Dad will be in from work soon and you had better all behave." We were all handed a sugar sandwich, after lunch Nan told me to go into the front room and watch out of the window to see if Dad was coming. I told her that I wasn't allowed to go in there because it had a broken window and it was Mum's room, but she just whacked me around the head and told me to do as I was told. I walked up the hallway I didn't want to go in Mum's room all I could think about was when the two men had been in there, I ran back to the Kitchen and stood in the doorway. "Well?" she shouted! "I" "I" "I'm not allowed in there Nan" I stuttered. Nan then took off her shoe and hit me with it and shouted "now get in there and do what you are told" I started to cry and turned back up the Hallway to Mum's room, my heart was racing and I was shaking as I opened the door slowly. I didn't know what to expect and I hesitated before I slowly walked in. I saw that Mum's bed had gone and there was no sign of her ever being in there at all. I was disappointed I wondered where Mum was. Nan shouted through "Well have you looked yet?" "I'm just going" I replied, she shouted back "I haven't got all day now move yourself child." I hurried over to the window and stood on the chair and looked out but all I could see was old man Bill picking up all the fag dog ends that he found on the floor, that he would then use to make roll-ups with, I also saw Mrs B's Family. I got back down and rubbed my backside which was stinging where Nan had whacked me I shut Mum's door and ran back to the Kitchen area I told Nan nervously that I hadn't seen him and she asked me if I had actually looked I said "that I had" and told her that I had seen old man Bill and Mrs B's Family she said "oh did you now well you had better sit on that chair and don't move you are going to cop it when your Dad gets in". I didn't understand what I had done wrong I had only done what she had told me to do, by now I was crying very loudly and she shouted at me that it was no good me crying. I went and sat on the sofa too afraid to move. Then the door opened and in walked Dad "What is she crying for?" he asked Nan "she went into the room with the broken window so I gave her a whack" lied Nan "you what" he said as he pulled me off the sofa and smacked me, I cried "she told me to" as I pointed at Nan "Oh a bloody liar am I" she said, with that he pulled me towards the stairs "now get up there and no dinner for you" he shouted "I did as I was told" I said as I went up the stairs. I fell on my bed and cried my backside really hurt, I got changed in to my pyjamas and shouted down "I hate you, I want my Mum!" I then cried myself to sleep.

The next day we went back to our usual school, Point school, the teacher asked if I had liked it at the other school I said "I didn't liked the new school", and didn't say much too any one that day, I was missing mum to much. I don't remember who picked us up that day but I do remember going in doors and all of us being frozen to the spot as we saw a woman sat on the sofa with a baby on her lap, I had seen this woman before but I couldn't remember where. Dad told us to all made stand in a line Youngest to Eldest and then said "Your mothers gone, this is your new mum and you will call her mum if I hear you lot calling her anything other than Mum you will have my toe up your arse, is that clear", then he told us the baby was called Debs. No one dared to say a word, I couldn't understand why she was in our house I wanted to know where Mum was. Most of us would speak in whispers about Mum, we were too scared to speak out loud, I would look at the place on the wall where her photo used to be and wonder where her apron had gone. All her belongings were gone and this new woman's stuff was in our house, placed were mums things once stood.

She had been moved in. We all missed our Mum so much and knew that life would never be the same without her. The first night with this new woman in Mums house was horrible, as the days went we were calling her Bumble, when no one was about to hear us, she never said much to us at that time, but the looks she gave to us all scared me, scared us all. After tea we were soon sent off to bed whether it was nearly time for bed or not. As we all went to give our Dad a kiss as we would have to do normally, Bumble pointed to the stairs and said "bed" we said "we haven't kissed our dad yet" she said "you don't need to do that, that all ends now". We didn't understand what she meant but we didn't argue we just went up to bed. She didn't like us and as the days went on she made it quite clear she didn't. As the time went on I remembered where I had seen Bumble before she had been the woman that had asked Roy and I for Dad while we were outside the house and she was the same woman that Mum and I had seen with Dad the day Mum said that we were playing, Hide and Seek and saw Dad. Bumble would often tell me that I should have gone with Mum, and I used to wish that I had. She had no intention of being a nice to us. The happy house that Mum had made for us all changed the day Bumble moved in. One day she told us she was getting rid of Mum's beloved cats Sleepy and Ben, I cried out "why?" she said to me "you mind your own business you ugly cow it's nothing to do with you" she poked her finger in my face and gave me one of her evil looks, she took great pleasure in seeing that I was upset "now get out of my sight" she said. I ran to the toilet outside and cried I then heard her calling so I wiped my face and went into the Kitchen she then ordered me to bed, I didn't even look up I just went. The next day I asked Lizzie where Sandy was "she doesn't come round anymore" I said "shhhhh" said Lizzie "she might hear you" she said, meaning Bumble. I felt scared and I missed my big Sister but I missed Mum more. A few days later we came home from school and were all shocked to see that the entire house had been packed up and all that was left was the sofa in the sitting area, we were told to sit on the sofa and told not to move. It was cold sitting there as the fire hadn't been lit, we were handed a sugar sandwich and told not to make a mess. We all looked at each other and we saw the fear in each others eyes but no one said a word. Silent tears ran down my face. Late that night we were all put in the van, by that time I was half asleep we then drove away. It didn't seem that we had driven very far when the van stopped and we were told to get out quickly and quietly. We were taken into a house that was cold damp and smelly. We were given a blanket to share and had to cuddle up together on a sofa to go to sleep. Ollie and Jake had to stay up and help. The next morning we woke up and realised with the light now shining in that we were in a dismal room. We were all shivering with cold and hungry, no one said a word we just looked at each other and looked around the room. Next our Dad came in and said "the toilets in the garden which is down the hall, into the kitchen and out the back door and to the left" he then went back out of the room into the Kitchen where I could hear him talking to The Thing Off the living room, where we had spent the night was the front door which was opposite the stairs. Under the stairs there was a cellar, which we were told not to go in. I hated it as did the others we all wanted to go home, we were taken upstairs and shown to our rooms. Here we were with Dad and Bumble and no Mum, the pets had all gone including Sleepy and Ben. I noticed that my favourite doll was missing. My main concern at that time was Mum I worried about where she was and I was concerned that she wouldn't know that we had moved and wondered how she would find us. I couldn't ask where my Mum was as I was too scared to say anything to Bumble as I remember asking where the pets were and she had slapped me round the face and had told me to shut up. I was scared and upset my Mum would never have done anything like that.

To us when it got too much I would sit and hide behind a chair and cry quietly for my Mum so that Bumble couldn't see or hear me, I became so terrified of Bumble, but every time someone knocked on the door my heart would race I would think that it was Mum and that she had found us at last but every time I was to be disappointed when it wasn't her. Every night I prayed Mum would come and find us. Bath time became a nightmare time, I grew to hate the mention of bath time, even in mid winter I was put into a bath full of cold water, and there was no fire on. Bumble would hold my hair and put my whole head under the water she would bring me back up so I could gasp for another breath and then she would hold me back under all the time laughing and sneering. I was too petrified to complain for fear that she would hold me under and not let me up for breath. When I got out of the bath she would open the back door wide so that I had to stand there in the cold, naked and shivering. My teeth would chatter together and I would have goose bumps all over my body. While I got dressed she would slap me and flick my ears while calling me names and laughing, when she was bored with that she would push me up the Hallway where I could then to go into the Living room where at least it was warmer as the fire would be glowing. I couldn't understand why she would treat me like this. I remember when Mum used to give me a bath; she would hang the towels over a chair near the fire so that they could be warming up. She would check the temperature of the water with her elbow to check that it was nice and warm. She would then gently pour the water over my head to wash my hair when I was washed she would lift me out and wrap a nice warm towel around me and gently rub me dry and quickly get me dressed for bed so that I wouldn't get cold. She would then brush my hair through, if I screamed out that it was pulling with the knots she would say "Sorry love nearly done."

Then one day Bumble called me out to the Kitchen and said "do you want any breakfast?" "Yes please" I replied "well it's in the bin so you had better get it out" she said with an evil laugh. I looked at her and then looked at the bin, I started to cry and said to her "I can't eat that it's all dirty" with that she grabbed me by the hair and dragged me to the bin where she grabbed a handful of dirty rotten food and shoved it in my mouth, I spat it out and started screaming. She started shouting "eat it you ugly Bitch." My Dad then came in the room wanting to know what all the noise was about and Bumble looked at him and said "the little Bitch has just threw her breakfast all over the floor" "you what!" he said as he slapped and pushed me "she's lying" I said "don't you dare lie to me now clear it up now" my Dad shouted back, all the while hitting and pushing me, he then left the room. As soon as he had Bumble grabbed me by the hair and said to me with a sneer "no one will believe you, you ugly shit, you are a worthless piece of shit", she then pushed me to sink and said "now clean up before I call your Dad." As I bent down to clean up with a cloth I was crying with the pain of the whacks my dad had just given me, Bumble then came up behind me, put her foot on my back and pushed me over onto the floor and told me to get out of her sight. She then left the Kitchen to go into the Living room when I had finished cleaning up I started walking towards the Living room where I heard Bumble shouting and Paul crying, Paul then ran up the stairs holding his head I asked Roy what Paul had done wrong and he said that Paul hadn't done anything wrong Bumble had just started hitting him around the head for no reason. None of us understood why she was so nasty and cruel to all of us, Dad seemed to believe everything she said and she used to make sure he gave us a beating for things that we hadn't even done. One day when I was thinking about Mum and crying to myself because I missed her so much Bumble called me to her and said "why are you crying?" "I miss my mum" I said "oh miss you're Mum do you, well your Mums gone, she never loved you that's why I'm here." "I don't believe you Mum does love us she told us all the time" I cried and ran out to the back garden and sobbed. Later I tried to tell Dad what Bumble had said but he wouldn't believe me and hit me for lying. Soon it was Christmas 1963 I was nine years old and I wrote a letter to Santa saying Dear Santa, I just want Mummy to come and find us, I don't want anything else for Christmas, just my Mum, I folded it up and put it up the chimney. I remember hoping that Santa would answer my letter or that he would bring Mum to come and get us. When I didn't get a reply a few days later I wrote another letter as I was about to throw it up the chimney Bumble saw it and snatched it out of my hand she read it out loud "Dear Santa!, you aren't getting anything" she sneered and then she threw it on the open fire where it burned, I started to cry "have something to cry about" she said, as she smacked me around the head. If any one tried to comfort me they would have been hit to for interfering.

No one dare try to comfort any one of us when one had been laid into it just made things worse, as much as everyone wanting to help. Bumble would love to see us cry and usually after she had made us cry she would then leave us alone because she had achieved what she wanted. I actually now believed I was worthless, In private we would comfort each other and said sorry to each other for not helping at the time but we all knew it was the only way we could deal with things if we had interfered we would have got a belting and the one originally getting the beating would get hit twice as hard, we just had to learn to cope by ourselves.

I tried to help Roy once with his chore of filling up the coal bucket, the bucket was too heavy for him so when he had picked it up the coal had spilt out I had rushed to help him scoop it back in the bucket when Dad had grabbed me by the neck of my jumper and the seat of my trousers and had slung me out the door and out into the Hallway. "Who asked you to interfere?" he shouted while hitting me "Go to bed" he shouted at me while I ran as fast as I could up the stairs to get away from him. From my bed I could hear him hitting and shouting at Roy he was shouting at him "you are a useless Bastard you can't do anything right." And then I heard Bumbles voice "gone on Ed you give him what for" she was taking pleasure in Roy's suffering as she did with us all, I just hid under my covers and covered my ears with my pillow and cried.

Chapter 4

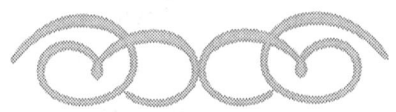

New Year New horrors

As a new year began, I never gave up hope of mum finding us I refused to believe anything Bumble said she hated us all and it showed in all she did and said and the way she treated us, I became confused by time, so I knew my months by birthdays, and kept track that way! My eldest sister had taught me them.

January came and went with no sign of mum but I wasn't giving up hope that she would find us and take us home to the life we knew.

I hated dad, Bumble and the house in which we were living, we all did but we had to survive this life of hell.

Some of my siblings went to the local school at the top of the road the elder ones to the local secondary school. I enjoyed school it was better than being at home with Dad and Bumble, I hated weekends and school holidays those times were even worse, not just for me but for us all.

I enjoyed school it was better than being at home with them, those times were even worse, under her feet as she would call it, we made her blood boil as she often reminded us just to look at us she would say.

At school half term approached she knew how we felt about holidays, she would rub her hands together and say "God help ya."

As half term came she started taunting me telling me I was ugly, I was a waste of space she gloated, as I cried and then told me "you are going wish you died with mother you ugly little shit" Those words rang round my head "Died with Ya mother" I cried even more I was so upset I screamed at her "my mum was coming back for me!" The look of pure evil was on her face she was enjoying every minute of it I was so upset i went back at her again, "you're evil and cruel and I hate you" I could hear my heart racing pounding like it was going to burst from beneath me. "Not as much as I hate you lot" she bellowed back at me. "Your mum an't coming back she's dead" "NO" I sobbed. She had said it and meant it!

I ran to my dad through the sobs I cried "she said my mum was dead! "She's not is she?" I sobbed.

He starred fixed on me then said "yes six feet under of course she died you silly cow."

My whole world just stopped for that split second it just stopped my heart beating faster I sobbed uncontrollably. I ran as fast as my feet could carry me out the door down the street the buildings moved faster than they had ever moved. I carried on till I reached the bottom of the road to derelict ground. I hid and sobbed and sobbed the realisation that my mums yes my mum was never coming back, my mum had died!

I felt like someone had ripped my heart out id never felt hurt like it, I wanted to wake up and it all be a dream a horrible dream. But it wasn't a dream it was real very, very real.

The dream my mum would come and fetch us sweeps us up in her loving arms gone!

I felt sick my whole body shaking as I sobbed I screamed out "MUM WHY."

Someone suddenly grabbed my arm, "love what's wrong, look at the state of you, I could hear you sobbing, what is so wrong tell me" as she pulled me towards her she put her arm around me, "there there" she said "calm you're self down, tell me what's upset you" Through the sobbing I managed to tell her " my mum is dead, she's never coming back" I cried even more she put her arm round and pulled me close for a cuddle "I'm so sorry love you poor little dear don't cry, Ya mum will always be watching over you and will always love you as much as she ever did."

I could have stayed there forever that warmth of a cuddle that meant something. Like the cuddle mum gave so often when we were upset or feeling blue or just for being me.

It was as if mum were there comforting me then I realised this wasn't mum. My mum's cuddles were like no other and I'd never have that again.

The woman lead me away from the derelict ground "come on love" she said, she obviously knew me. She led me home. The woman knocked on the door still with her arm around me comforting me. The door swung open and there stood Bumble "where have you been" she shouted at me. The woman briefly explained how upset I was to learn that my mother had died. Bumble Just grabbed me by the arm through the door and hit me knocking me to the floor.

"Did you not hear the child has just heard her mother has died and is upset" begged the woman. Bumble moved towards the woman and said "Do I look fucking dead, she's a little shit." She slammed the door in the woman's face.

I knew that I was in trouble what did they care I was upset the tears streamed down my face still sobbing, I can't be hurt any more than I had already.

I could hear Bumble shouting down the cellar to dad screaming at him about what had happened at the door. Suddenly I could hear his steps coming closer and closer he pushed passed Bumble and grabbed me! I prepared myself for what was to come. I could feel the rigidness of the fear through out my body.

"What are you trying to do" Dad was screaming directly at my face could feel his Bellows on my face, he layed into me thud thud thud blow after blow. "Get to your bed and stay there" I turned to run up the stairs and he rained one last kick as I hit the stair. I ran up them stairs as fast my legs would carry me.

I ran through into my bedroom and climbed straight into my bed. I could Feel emptiness inside me!

I lay on the bed sobbing not because of the kicking or the laying into me, that didn't hurt like the words that my beloved dearest mum was dead that's what hurt more than any kicks or blows or slander. They didn't even care they might as well have ripped out my heart!

Now more than anything I wanted my mum nobody else could make this better. The realisation that I was not going to see that beautiful person again was the hardest thing to bear. I even questioned whether it was just a horrible joke the ones Bumble had fun with. But I realised quite quickly the sheer hatred in Bumbles face she enjoyed every darn moment of it. She enjoyed the horror on my face she enjoyed the fact that she was the one to tell me she enjoyed the fact that I was hurting. Me I hated Bumble more than anything why did my mum die she was a good kind person I don't think id ever understand why!

Again I had to miss dinner, what had I done that was so wrong, I could not understand it, it was worse here, by the time Lizzy had come to bed, I had calmed myself down and pretended to be asleep. I didn't want to speak to anyone encase I started to cry again and what if she didn't know the truth about our mum, our beautiful loving mum. I missed her more than ever knowing she was never coming back.

Next morning my eyes were still swollen from the crying, I could hear my name being called it was Bumble she was calling me to get down stairs.

As I approached the kitchen she shouted at me "eat that" she handed me last nights dinner just as I reached to take it she pulled the plate back took a deep breath then spat on it before thrusting it in my face. "Eat it or else" she snarled at me with that wicked glare on her face. I sat looking at the plate not even the absolute emptiness of my stomach could bring me to lift the fork.

I could not bear to eat it; I wouldn't eat it the thought of what she had done made me heave. But lunch time came and she again handed me the same dinner again withdrawing it from me to spit on it then thrusting it back at me to eat. I couldn't I wouldn't it was given to me again at dinner same routine withdrawn and spat in before thrusting it at me. I decided I would take handfuls of food to the toilet discreetly and put it down the loo until the dinner had gone, and I'd say id been sick if anyone asked. I'd just realised this was survival time!

Before we knew it it was 1964, I was coming up nine now. No one was allowed to even kiss dad goodnight not even Debs was allowed now. In fact life for Debs became like our Life it got harder and cruel. No one at this time was sure if our dad was Debs dad.

Yet the curtain never moved for Debs either, we all knew why Bumble hated us and egged dad on. Not that he needed much help. We came to the understanding, he would do anything to keep her, we often heard the rows and she would threaten to leave him, we all became aware and most understanding to the Abusive Life we had come accustomed to. We all were trying to survive. And wonder each day would we survive.

It didn't take much to think back to when mum was alive, her cuddles and love the warmth of her smile the happier times when she was here with us. This memory of mum was our way to survive this evil and cruel life.

Just to think of that smile warmed my heart up inside it had been along time since any of us smiled. I wished for her cuddles sometimes wishing so hard I could feel them her warm arms wrapped around me.

Dad became a Brut a real monster, I'd always remember when mum was alive how he reduced her to tears, he would hit us and belt us at a young age, mum hated it, always trying to protect us, but he was never the monster he had become.

We held on to the memories of the golden years and the thought of finding our eldest sister, whom we were not allowed to mention. I remember sitting there wishing that it was he who died and not our mum things were so different.

But soon another school term came to an end just the thought of being at home sent dread into me. At the end of July we were told school was out for six weeks. I remember the teacher asking each of us what we would be doing she went around each child in the class. Then it was my turn I sat in silence, what I had to look forward to! "Surely there is something you're doing a big adventure maybe" said the teacher in excitement "none that I know of miss" I replied "may be visit Ya grandparents" "no I don't think so miss," I replied, you could see the look on her face she was desperately trying to think of ideas "Maybe visit your Mummies parents" I replied very soberly "No I don't think so, they are dead like my mum," "Ow my you mustn't say horrible things like that" she quickly replied " but it is true miss" I said, but before she could reply the bell rang out and everyone jumped to there feet to leave the classroom.

As I got up to leave the teacher stopped me "Miss Barker you have a very wild imagination and if you say things like that in class you could find yourself in a lot of trouble" she said sympathetically. I looked up at her and told her "it's true all of it my mum was dead and I didn't know my grandparents, I think they were dead too, im not lying miss" She looked slightly alarmed, "Well who is that woman that came to the school not so long ago she's your mum surely" "She's not my mum miss; she's not you ask my brothers she's not my mum". I wanted her to understand that I was telling the truth but she just patted me on the head and told me to run along and go and enjoy my holiday and stop inventing stories. Why didn't she believe me it was true.

As I waited for my brothers outside the school gate, the teacher passed and smiled and said "you are a funny girl, there are all the other children here glad to be on holiday and here you are rather be at school." She then turned walked away then looking back said "you are a mystery my girl" the thoughts ran through my head I wanted to shout them from the roof tops. If only that teacher knew if she had to go home to what we do you'd rather be at school, this was my safety net our only place we could escape the troubles of home.

Little did I know the teacher had been telling Bumble and my dad what I had said in school as she was worried about my imagination running wild! This only made things worse for me.

The weeks passed most days we were kicked out in to the street weren't allowed to knock for a wee or a drink. Some days we were only allowed in if she demanded, we used to go up to the derelict grounds to wee hoping we wouldn't get caught. When we weren't kicked out on to the street we were made to do chores all day like little slaves god helps us if we didn't do them. We had no toys, bikes or prams as the other children in the street had. We all spent some of our time sitting on the pavement watching them all playing. We made up games to play to keep ourselves amused; we'd throw stones in the air and catch them on the backs of our hands. By tea time we were very hungry we were given a jam sandwich and half cup tea. It was always the same never any variety.

There were lots of things we never understood, no one knew why and was not allowed to question, but there was a lot of whispering that went on, and dad went into hospital. While he was in hospital that week was hell because she was now free to commit whatever abuse she felt. We became slaves at her beck and call regardless what anyone of us did it was never good enough; she just wanted any excuse to hit, punch and kick us. She was like a cat that had her cream and she was enjoying it. She would have us all in tears with her evil tongue. This for as hard as it became for us was an everyday abusive circle. She said so many horrible things, things that were so cruel and hurtful; she would call us by horrible pet names. Sometimes the things she said were more hurtful than the beatings. She accused us of allsorts. We all learnt really quickly that there was no point in crying that just made her worse and harder reigns on us. Some times when dad would use the buckle end of the belt to attack us she would have a grin on her face ear to ear.

If one of us were about to cry we all did our best to silence them because we knew that we all in turn be punished in some way for the tears they shed.

We were banned from certain parts of the house like the cellar and shop. She ordered us to do things and we learnt just to do whatever no questions just do it.

When we visited him in hospital she would gloat about how bad we all had been, we tried to defend ourselves, I mean we daren't be naughty or disobedient we knew what we would get off her. But he wouldn't listen it made no difference he believed her every time. She would lean towards him and look at us from the corner of her eyes. He wasn't bothered about us he just wanted to see her. She loved it loved every minute. At home a bucket was placed on the landing of a night to wee in that was what we had been reduced to.

If any of us tried to use the toilet out back of the garden she would knock us about and make it quite clear where our toilet was. This repulsed me she wasn't even prepared to share a toilet with us. But the one thing I hated more than anything was bath times it was my nightmare and it got no better with each bath time, no matter how much I prepared myself. I dreaded the word alone. She'd push my face in the water holding it down and watch me struggle for air the dreaded taunts, the hair pulling. The thought of it made me feel sick my heart would pound with the fear. There was times when she washed me down with Vim or carbolic soap that was her favourite bath torture. She would scrub and scrub at my skin until it was red and bleeding. I would just close my eyes wish away the time the pain would turn numb just for a few seconds. Then the realisation would hit me the pain unbearable I held back the tears cause I knew that if I was dare to cry this could be worse than it already was.

She'd cook meals the most disgusting meals I truly cannot remember a descent dinner with that woman it was always the same meals potatoes and slice bread or potatoes spam and half a tomatoes, there were times she gave us a plate of broken biscuits another was bread and sugar. Their meals were cooked separate to ours. She invented stories to tell dad and we knew and she knew that when he got home we would cop it so we dreaded that day. She was so cock sure of herself she'd have that smirk on her face, them eyes glaring at you. She often didn't need to open her mouth the looks said it all. It would send the fear of god into you, but her well she enjoyed every bit of it watching us with fear in our faces. She would get great pleasure from watching us squirm.

I used to have terrible nightmares and Bumble would say it was the "devil" after me, and that I had bad dreams because I was going to an evil place, because I was an evil kid. I believed her why wouldn't I, I was just a child. I became scared of the dark. We never understood why she did what she did what had we done so badly! My thoughts always went back to my mum and the happiness she spread I could feel the security of her almost like she was there she always made us feel safe, my mum loved us so much and told everyday you would see the pride in her eyes. But Bumble she didn't know what the word love was, she didn't know how to love she was not capable of showing love. She was the most heartless woman we were ever to come across in our life and one that we become to hate, yes hate even at the age I was I couldn't stand this woman I hated her for what she had done to our lives. My brother would whisper to me that she was the devil!

Bumble would take us to visit dad I remember one occasion, it was a lovely sunny day as we arrived he was sitting on a bench outside the grounds. He was so pleased to see her but told us all to take a walk. We did as we were told and strolled around but we were stopped by a doctor and told we had to return to our dad.   As we arrived back to where we had left dad and Bumble they weren't on the bench. But then we heard noises coming from the bushes, we all took a look and found dad had his trousers round his ankles, and she had her knickers round her ankles and her skirt to her waist. We were horrified at what we had seen; I didn't really understand what they were up too. But Bumble shouted to go away. I never really understood what was happening until I over heard the elder ones talking about it, and how disgusted they had been by it all. Then I sort of understood. I remember Roy saying "I suppose we all dreamt that to." We all laughed at Roy's remark because that was just typical of what she would say. I remember over hearing a conversation that dad was in a Psychiatric hospital. At the time I never understood what that meant, but as I got older I realised the meaning. Well eventually dad came home and made up for lost time he layed into some of us over things Bumble had said we had done. She stood there laughing enjoying every minute of it knowing that it was all untrue, but we didn't even have the strength to argue.

Bumble became worse not wanting us to smile, laugh or have any fun. My brother pulled a face behind her back once I remember she reached out and grabbed us for laughing slapping us furiously round the face or arm " what you laughing at you ugly shit" she would scream "nothing" I said. Then she slapped me again saying "see if that's funny" as she was Snarling at me. She couldn't stand us laughing she would attack whoever she found laughing. One of her favourite tricks was to slap us with a wet hand the imprint of her hand would imprint on our bodies. She would grab you arms and twist the skin like a Chinese burn. The look of pure pleasure was etched on her face at every attack. The more you cried the more she inflicted so we tried so hard not to cry knowing if we did it would last longer.

We didn't see so much of dad as he spent much of his time in the cellar making furniture to sell. If he wasn't working days then he would work nights.

So we would be slung in the street by Bumble and warned not to come back for a wee or a drink.

Then she'd tell us all to get in of an evening and make us do all the chores around the house.

Other days we spent all day cleaning over and over until she was satisfied. Then order us all to bed by 6pm so we were out of her way.

I remember quite clearly that the days we were kicked to the street the neighbour's kids would taunt us, then dad would come charging out of the house and make us fight them. None of us had a violent streak in us despite all we went through. This particular day he ordered me to go and hit one of the Clarke girls, I couldn't do it, he grabbed me by the arm and threw me in the road "get over there before I bloody hit you" he shouted. I scrambled to my feet trying to tend to my grazed knee but he shouted "NOW" I just couldn't do it I couldn't hit her. The next thing I knew he came at me and hit me around the face knocking me to the ground. As I cried he shouted "hit her or I will hit you again" all the neighbours kids looking on in absolute amazement at what was happening to me. I knew that if I didn't want another hiding I would have to hit the girl, so I ran towards her and smacked her face apologising at the same time "harder you silly cow, hit her again" he bellowed at me. The poor girl at this stage was in total shock as I took another swoop at her apologising again before running back to the road side. Suddenly dad grabbed me and hit me the hardest he had ever hit me I went flying to the ground "that's a hit you silly cow" he screamed at me. He then turned to Lizzie and ordered her to go and fight with the eldest of the Clarke girls like me she couldn't bring herself to hit her. He ordered Lizzie again, she nervously walked over to the Clarke girl and stood looking at her, Lizzie was crying she couldn't` hit her. Dad was getting really angry at this point because she wouldn't comply. He shouted at her going red in the face with anger, he then unstrapped his belt. Poor Lizzie the fear showed in her face she hesitated as to what to do. I ran quickly in the house and out the back, thorough the alley to where my sister was but where dad couldn't see me. I called to the Clarke girl still listening to dad screaming at Lizzie to hit her or else, she came forward as Lizzie followed her, I gave her the hardest clump I could and another really layed into her for all the taunts she had done to us in the past. I pulled up Lizzie's top and ruffled her hair then ran back through the house and stood beside dad "where have you been" he said "to the toilet dad" I replied. The Clarke girl was really screaming and ran home, Lizzie came running towards dad he started laughing "you can do it when I threaten Ya" This is what we were reduced to just to survive the abuse from Bumble and dad.

Next thing the Clarke girls dad came marching over "what's your bloody problem making these kids fight each other" before he could finish what he was saying dad attacked him one huge punch and the bloke was lying there on his back. Dad brushed his hands and ordered us all inside as he followed us.

After that not many kids would play with us knowing what dad was like.

Our elder sister Jane worked and we were told she was not to be told about what happened during the day. We knew not to tell either because we knew what we would end up with. But we were always pleased to see Jane when she return from work, always got a hug and a kiss even to that Bumble face told all by the looks she gave. Jane had a horrible life with dad and Bumble too, they were so nasty to her we use to get really upset and cry to see what she went through and how she sobbed at the abuse she received. Her job was her sanity she couldn't wait to leave the house and who could blame her, but at the same time she did not want to leave us, but she had to work to keep her self as they made clear to her.

Not one day of the school holidays were fun, we used to make up our own games I remember one of the neighbours giving us a skipping rope and we were delighted but as soon as Bumble saw it she took it away.

The weeks past in which we were glad about we wished the weeks away so we could get back to school.

Everyday became so routine with the abuse, kicks, punches the taunts they all came our way. The chores were our jobs while Bumble screamed at us to do it prompt god help us if they weren't.

One particular night after the bath time horrors I was sent to the living room the telly was on, and I heard the words bank holiday and knew that our holidays were nearly over. I repeated what I had heard to the others, suddenly Bumble came charging in and accused me of putting on the telly, but that was just another excuse to lay into me and that she did. She screamed at me to get to my room it wasn't even worth arguing I just went crying to my room. She made me miss tea again that night. The nights were still light so I read a comic belonging to Jake and drifted off to sleep. When I awoke it was dark and Lizzie was asleep. I could feel the urge for a wee so crept out to the landing to use the bucket, someone has done a number two in the bucket, and so I squatted over did my wee and headed back to my room. Suddenly Bumble called me "what are you doing out of bed" I looked at her, "I done a wee in the bucket" She came out to the landing looked into the bucket then suddenly turned slapping me "that bucket is for pissing in not shitting you dirty cow" she bellowed I started to cry then she hit me again get to your room I'll sort you out in the morning.

I couldn't sleep afraid of what she would do in the morning in the morning I was called down to the living room. Dad was standing there staring at me I knew by that glare that I was in trouble "I heard that you went a poo in the bucket last night" he said really calmly I looked up at him surprised at no raised voice, "no dad I did a wee in the bucket that's all" "so you are calling Bumble a liar then are you" he said with a sudden change in his voice. "Yes she is" I replied nervously, he turn`t to Bumble and said "she said you're a liar".

She got out of the chair towards me with a clenched fist I stepped back towards dad and fell on him, he grabbed my arm and hit me before pushing me towards Bumble I could feel the punches in my back as she reined the blows then she ordered me to clean out the bucket. I could feel the intense pain in my back I was sobbing in pain. I picked myself up and left the living room to clean out the bucket. The others were all up and about by this time and breakfast were underway. Bumble asked me if I was hungry I told her eagerly that I was, she turned her back then came at me with a plate of scraps which were left over scraps from the previous night, Bumble spat on it then demanded that I eat all of it. I went into the living room I lay it on the arm of the chair and went out to the toilet and got handfuls of tissue, I then wrapped the food up in it and discreetly made several trips to the toilet until it was all gone.

Before we knew it school was upon us and I was so excited I couldn't sleep the night before through excitement.

The next morning we were all up early washed and dressed, Lizzie done breakfast and made sure I had a good meal Eight thirty came and we were all sent out the door to school that was after a warning that we were to make excuses for the bruises if anyone was to ask. As the door shut behind us we started to walk up the road to school, I noticed Lizzie crying and asked her what was wrong. " look at my shoes everyone at school are going to take the mickey out of me not that they need a excuse" she sobbed, I looked down at her shoes she had a pair of dads old shoes on, they were tied around her feet to keep them on with string. "What shall I do" she sobbed. I had an idea I quickly run back home banged on the door as it opened I pushed passed and run up the stairs. I grabbed Lizzie's plimsolls and stuffed them in my satchel before running back out and up the street to Lizzie. I handed her the Plimsolls and agreed where we would meet on the way home that evening so she could change back in to the old shoes of dads. She kissed and hugged me she was so pleased and then we went our separate ways to school. School was good that day but it was over too soon and before we knew it the bell was ringing out for home time. I meet up with Lizzie and she changed over her plimsolls for the old shoes. We headed home and I headed straight upstairs so I could hide her plimsolls and get changed. Once I had done that I headed down stairs just as Lizzie had come in. This happened over several days just so she didn't get teased about the shoes. But day's later dad had managed to find out what I had been doing for Lizzie he hit me so hard I nearly passed out! I told him it was all my idea and that Lizzie had nothing to do with it thankfully he only warned her. But it was worth it knowing how relieved Lizzie felt knowing she wasn't being bullied at school no more than she already was.

We were all told to be in bed early at six thirty in the evening, little did Bumble know I enjoyed going to bed it meant I was out of their company. I remember 1966 was the world cup and England beat Germany everyone was out in the street except us we just had to listen to the cheers from inside.

It was not long after that we were told we would be moving everyone was piled into the back of the van, the journey started to see our new house. After a while we pulled up outside this house but we were told to stay in the van. So we only got a glimpse of the outside of the house. Weeks later a van pulled up outside and Haggie and dad started to load up with boxes of stuff, but only certain things were being put into the van, when I suddenly realised it was all Jane's stuff they were slinging her out, we all cried for days it broke our heart she was so upset, we were told in no uncertain terms that we were not to have any contact with her. It was so unfair she had done nothing wrong yet was thrown out to fend for herself.

We were told we would be moving to the new house soon, and it would be goodbye to Starling Way and our schools and be off on another journey wondering what would lie ahead!

Chapter 5

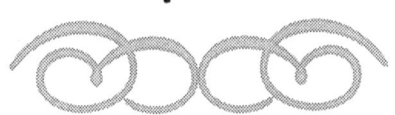

LITTLE SLAVES

*M*y brothers and sisters and I hoped a new house a new beginning, but our eyes told us not to expect too much.

Jane had been kicked out of starling way, while living there her life became a misery of threats and abuse and the name calling with dad and Bumble. Jane worked in a factory, off to work she went as normal kissed us goodbye. To return home to her belongings all thrown in the back of a van, still not understanding why they did this we tried to question why this had happened but dad and

Bumble told us to it didn't concern us. Although we knew it did.

I can recall that day so well. That was the Last time we saw Jane for years to come. When at home in Cellars rd, when mum was alive Jane was like mums shadow never left her side, mum used to say "why don't you go out side with the others, instead of being cooped up in here?" but Jane would reply "I'm ok here with my book mum," knowing   Jane never wanted to be away from mum, a lot of Jane's reasons were because she was trying to protect mum from dad. Jane having been kicked out had made a lot of impact to our lives as big sister, she gave us love and comfort, Jane begged them to let her stay, but they would not hear of Jane's plights.

None of us knew why or where Jane would go, we were not allowed to mention her name, no more than we were allowed to mention Sandy's, but it never stopped us thinking about them, that night most of us cried we knew this was Bumble's fault. Bumbles aggression and abuse became worse her tongue evil. Jake seemed to escape the physical abuse he was stronger than all of us but she did abuse him verbally but Jake seemed to stand up for himself some how. In the school holidays Lizzie had to take us out to the local park some days to get out of their hair as they put it, no food no drink   we she weren't allowed to take us home until tea time, it would be home tea and bed, if you were lucky to get any tea. Lizzie was given full responsibility of us younger ones, if anything happened she would get a belting for not watching us, if for some reason we played up she would have to tell them, if she didn't and they found out she and us would be in big trouble, but either way it caused resentment between us. It was all to survive. Other days we had to play out front of the house or do chores, depending on her moods she was very unpredictable was Bumble.

Soon the time came we were told we would be moving to a new area as the new house was now ready and we would all be attending new schools, I was not too happy about the school changing I was happy at the school I attended, but our opinions didn't count and no one dare say a word.

In days to come we started to pack up, we were not allowed to see inside the new house until the day of the move not knowing where we would be going, we would talk amongst our selves but dare not ask any questions regards to the move.

Finally the day came, we were not allowed to say goodbye to school friends or tell anyone of the move.

Off we went in the old van to start a new life in the new house we were all uneasy to where and what to expect the journey seemed long, the van stopped and we were all told to stay put while Bumble and dad entered in, all trying to look out the van windows to take view of the house as we tried to before, it looked more modern than the one we lived in, the turning was long, the school was about a 20 minute walk, A few local shops in which we had noticed not too far at the top of the road. Soon our father came out and let us out the van. We entered in the new house in Gates road. I was very happy as we where shown around this house noting it never had a cellar. We where shown our rooms all behind Bumble and dad we followed up the stairs. Lizzie and I had to share in which we were pleased about.

Our room was of fair size, and next to the inside bathroom and toilet which we were all pleased to see. Unfortunately the horrors began that night. Our hopes of a new house new beginning became short lived as I was soon to encounter.

I couldn't sleep properly that first night in the new house, strange place strange room, I got up to go to the toilet a little bewildered to where I was, feeling the wall as I walked slowly to feel for the light switch, next thing the light came on, and I was dragged by my arm by Bumble she began to hit me round the head, "what are you doing out of bed?"

She shouted at me," I wanted to go to the toilet I cried," "I'll give you bloody toilet" she claimed, as she still hit me around the head, "get in that bloody bed and don't you dare get out again" she said as she now slung me round on to my bed, "and if you wet your self god help you" she claimed leaving the room with that evil look upon her face.

I lay in bed crying and holding my self in hoping I wouldn't wet myself, afraid to sleep in case I did.

The night went slowly, seemed the morning was never coming, dying for the toilet, I really didn't think I could wait much longer, Why wouldn't she let me go I asked myself! I was petrified in case I wet myself.

As the time went it started to get light outside, I couldn't hold on any longer, my tummy hurting by now, I crept out on to the landing and crept to the toilet, in relief I just made it, I came out the toilet looking towards the stairs, as I was grabbed by the hair, "what did I bloody tell you, you little shit! Defy me would you" she shouted; as she pulled my hair dragging me back to my bed.

"You get out that bloody bed I'll break your neck" she claimed .I got under the covers and stayed there under my breath I was saying "I hate you."

As it became lighter out side I heard dads voice as he walked up the stairs, I heard his foot steps along the landing, next they seemed to get closer and stop, I heard his voice nearer, "I know you're awake you little bastard get up now" he demanded, no hesitating I got up, "down stairs now before you wake everyone." I hurried down stairs.

As I went into the kitchen she made a bee line for me, "what are you doing out of bed?" She said.

She sneered at me, as scared as I was I replied "dad told me to get up and get down stairs", she poked my face twisting her finger in my face so hard saying "if you're bloody lying god help you, you ugly bitch," with that dad came in, and ordered me to make the tea, and so I did.

I passed the tea to him with no thank you or anything he took the tea and ordered me to wash the dishes they had used during the night, I did with out question.

Soon my brothers and sisters were awake and came down Debs was hesitating to come in the kitchen.

We were given the orders for the day the many jobs that were to be done no one dare argue no one said a word; we were allowed to make a drink and were ordered to get dressed. We all just looked at each other.

To his commands we did as we were told, Up washed dressed, and back down.

Two had to unpack boxes with the kitchen items in and the living room items, two had to do the upstairs, and rest to help him in the garden to organise the shed stuff. In the living room Bumble was sat with her feet up, cup of tea in one hand fag in the other.

We were not allowed to stop until it was done as hungry as we were no one dare complain.

By now it was lunch time we had worked hard since 7am. I was ordered to run to the shop to get a loaf of bread, thankfully we had noticed where the shops were the day before, and so I was able to run there and back and not get a wallop for taking my time as dad or Bumble would say.

We were ordered to make a slice of toast for each of us not enough to feed our hunger but the toast and tea was made. Lizzie and I had to wash and dry the dishes and get back to the unpacking when we had finished the jobs down stairs, we had to go up and unpack the clothes.

As we unpacked, putting the clothes in piles I recalled the time our Jane had to go to the rag yard to buy our clothes, on dads demand. We never had nice things like new; some of the clothes we possessed were so tatty they were fit for the rag bag.

But I continued to do the job. Lizzie was called down stairs, as I unpacked I came across a jumper of Jane's and I held it close to me and began to cry, I missed her so much.

I wondered where she was, what she would be doing, was she in touch with sandy, I put her jumper on the top of my pile then hid it in the drawer with my things.

I kept it as a momentum and every night I retrieved this Jumper from my drawer and cuddled up to Jane's jumper for comfort. Within a few days we started our new schools, I went to Gates rd junior and Debs went to Gates rd infants, the others went to The Prêt School.

Home from school the first day neither was interested to know how we had all got on, tea that night was a plate of broken biscuits, for some reason as I went to sit I slipped and knocked the plate on the floor, dad shouted out "who's done that?" I owned up and claimed "I did dad," "get in here" she shouted, I went in to the living room, and before I could say sorry, I went flying across the room with one single punch from him, "It had to be you didn't it you little bastard" he shouted at me, I cried with the punch. I hit my head on the edge of the wall as I went down, then he shouted for me to get out of his sight as I made him feel sick.

I went back into the diner area and sat quiet "You alright?" the others whispered I nodded yes, I had to be no one dare come to my aid, or they would have got the same.

We were all called into the living room where we were told of our daily duties.

But it seemed we were to do everything No job for Bumble or dad to do, but that was nothing new, except spending money in the betting shop; she just gambled the money on bets on the dogs or horses. She certainly got her priorities right.

But we weren't surprised we were the little slaves. I was old enough now to know what was going on around us, and I understood more than they realised, well 7pm all to bed.

No one banked on staying there too long as if and when they wanted a cup of tea one of us had to get up and make it. I now truly believed this was all we were here for, to be there little slaves, at their beck and call.

Next morning we were all up to wash, dress, make the beds, do the breakfast if we were allowed, make a cup of tea, take them one up and then go back down to continue our jobs. Lizzie had to get the youngest one washed and dressed, I had to make all the beds, boys had to wash and dry up, floors had to swept and polished, kitchen floor washed, off to school we would go, leaving Lizzie to take the younger one to school then she would have to go back home to make them a fresh cuppa before she could continue on to school. Some days she attended school if other jobs needed doing, at lot of responsibility lie with Lizzie now as when before at the old house.

Jake was at work by now earning his own money, but he never seemed to stay at home much, once he got in he had a bath and out the door he went, but he had to put money in the meter to pay for his bath. Jake never bothered much about his dinner either then who could blame him; it wasn't worth coming home too. Some nights he never bothered coming home he spent some sleeping rough to avoid the torment. It wasn't long after Jake met a girl Ann Peters who he adored and she him. Ann was a lovely girl she came home to ours on many occasions and she would get upset at what she saw, there would be Lizzie up to her arm pits in washing using an old scrubbing board and a single tub washing machine that had to be filled with water, and an old mangle attached, having to put the clothes through by hand, in to the sink to rinse and then back through the mangle, it was hard work Lizzie was only 14 by now. The washing had to be hung out; this was my job to help. Ann offered to help Lizzie but Lizzie knew the consequences if Ann helped, Lizzie used to plead with Anne to go away while she carried out her jobs, encase Bumble or dad over heard this.

Soon Ann got to know what we had become accustomed to and how our father and Bumble worked. She too was scared of them.

It was around now that Debs was being taken away for days at a time but no one knew where or dare to ask, she would come home and be rather quiet and dad seemed to pick on her more often than he did before.

Ann was a lovely girl and she took a shine to us all, Debs took a real shine to her.

Jake and Ann became close, one day I recall them sitting on the settee cuddling up to each other, The Thing as Jake preferred to call her, accused them of having relations, she was jealous of Ann, and hated the thought of Jake happy.

Next thing we knew there were rows, and Jake had gone, Jake always helped us out, he gave us the money for our school needle work and cooking lessons to avoid the bullying from the teacher if we never had the money to pay. I recall Lizzie had the chance to go on a school trip; Dad said surprisingly she could go; Jake gave her money towards this every week. Lizzie brought stamps from the post office to save the money up, she had two and a half books of stamps worth £2-10s, a lot of money; and she discovered one day they were missing. Lizzie upset; dad asked what she was crying for she told him her saving books had gone missing for her school trip. We were all called in, stood in a line and he questioned each of us, like an interrogation parade, had us all crying, with his whacks and threats, Lizzie knew it was him that took them, across the road was a second hand shop where he bought rugs with the money he cashed the books in for. He was an evil so and so, put us through all that knowing he stole them.

The tables turned on Paul again, Bumble made his life a misery as dad did, and he was as bad as her. Paul missed Jake as they were buddies not just brothers. Jake was a musical person he had a guitar and would strum away to Elvis songs. Paul was called a streak of piss by Bumble, this upset Paul deeply, dad would taunt him with it to, like Jake, Paul was a nice looking lad, but Paul had became a nervous person which was not surprising the life he had, Paul used to wet the bed in fear, Lizzie and I used to try and help him by hiding the sheets till wash day or try an wash them in the bath if Bumble and dad went out. One particular day they discovered what was going on, and poor Paul he was made to walk up and down the street with a bill board on his back, that read   I WET THE BED! The kids in the street taunted him, Lizzie and I cried for him, of all the neighbours not one came to help him.

Paul was so upset at the way he was treated it made him more nervous.

Surviving this mental and physical abuse was a task in it self. Days and nights were So hard, some days I wondered how any of us would survive. I often wondered if I would be better off were mum was to get away from this abusive life, Bumble and dad loved playing the mind games with us all, on one occasion he was given a blue rug by a neighbour, he would ask one of us what colour it was, who ever would say blue, he would hit us and say it was green, so who ever would say it was green he would then hit us and say "don't you know green from bloody blue," or he would ask the shape of the rug, like he asked me, I said "oval". In which it was, He would say "its circle what is it?" I'd say "circle" so he would hit me and say "stupid cow its oval," no one could win with him. Screwing our minds up, we were all had a terrible life; we were all petrified of dad and Bumble. For some reason just out the blue Bumble started to take Debs away for a few days at a time as she had done for a while now but more often returning home in a foul mood. No one dare ask where she went or why.

Paul seemed to be picked on more so these days we were all picked on but Paul seemed to take the brunt of things now. He seemed to become the main target now, as weeks went by Paul was of age to leave school. Even that didn't help him.

She made his life a misery even before they discovered about the sheets, but when they did they made him lie in wet sheets, just humiliating him, in which Bumble got pleasure from.

The taunts got worse even though Paul was at work now he ended up leaving to go to do seasonal work, but not through choice. Even on his return home he was living a life of hell. In time he was gone too, just as the rest. Paul tried to bend over backwards to do right but it made no difference. My mums family were gradually going one by one, sandy wasn't allowed contact with us once mum died, then Jane kicked out then Jake now Paul. Lizzie and I cried for days, Roy he was always in endless trouble, not that he did anything, but they found any excuse for to lay into him as they did with any of us, but he was upset too that his brothers and sisters had gone and knew it was all Bumble and Dad's fault. Roy couldn't forgive them. It seemed strange that Debs was going away for days at a time and Paul was treated even worse, then Debs went never to return, we wondered had any of this had any bearing on the way she treated Paul worse. Missing and thinking of Paul I recall during a row with dad and Bumble we soon understood whatever had gone on Bumble did take it out on Paul more so. I over heard her say, soon after Debs had gone, "I won't see Debs again will I, and you're still not bloody satisfied" during the row dad said "and it weren't Paul's fault," "so bloody what, he pissed me off like they all do". She shouted back. Although the mystery of why Debs was gone no one knew, the mystery was still to be unfolded.

Lizzie was the target more so now having to stay home more than before, to clean and cook for them and do any shopping, just be at their beck and call as the slave. The school board was always coming round to the house, but some how dad always got away with it. The lies he told them were unreal. But after his visit Lizzie would have to return to school for a week or so.

At school I enjoyed netball, but was never allowed to stay after school for practice, it got to the stage I would deny he was my dad; I was so ashamed that people would think I was related to that. During a games lesson one day my teacher Mr Fen asked about the marks and bruises on my legs back and arms I said "I don't know" he looked at me and replied "so they just appeared over night then yes" I just stared at him, "how did you get the marks, I am asking you for the last time?" he was now shouting as I started to cry.

"My dad and stepmother did them I told him" through the tears, "right" he said "we are getting some where." He ordered the class to carry on with the bean bags.

He led me to the head teacher I was told to Stay there out side her office. Soon after they had a talk I was called in. "Right then" she said looking at my body, "your dad and stepmother did this to you yes?" She asked "yes" I replied.

"Ok wait outside for a moment please" she told me, as I walked out they started to talk. Then the door closed. I was sat there for some time Mr Fen returned back to the class.

Then to my horror there was dad, with that look on his face I had seen before, and I knew I was in for it.

He walked past me knocked on the head teacher's door, I started to shake, and I felt sick.

Why have they got him here? I asked my self holding back the tears.

The door opened, "In here now" I was ordered, I walked in slowly with my head down, "Yes miss" I said.

"You are going home with your father and will return tomorrow at 9am" she ordered.

Dad had a tight grip on my arm as he marched me up the corridor, towards the doors leading out of the school, he said "You just bloody wait till I get you home". He frog marched me up the road all the way home, swearing at me telling me I had disrespected him and that I was an ungrateful bitch, slapping me around the head.

We got closer to home, the closer we got the more I dreaded it, knowing what was to come. Soon we were home he opened the door pushed me inside, I fell to the floor he pulled me up by the hair and started kicking me and punching me, repeating his self about what an ungrateful little bitch I was and this was for telling lies, and had I anything to say for my self.

Amongst the sobs I said I had only told the truth as he had always told us to do.

He laid into me more, shouting "Don't you dare bloody patronise me," he took off his belt and belted me, curled up in a corner by now the belt just came my way repeatedly, across my backside.

"Well what you got to say for your self bitch?"

He screamed at me, I said "I've nothing to say".

He stopped belting me, grabbed me by the arm and locked me under the stairs. "You can bloody stay there you bitch, until you can apologise to me." He said I sat curled in a ball sobbing my eyes out, under the stairs, dark and scary.

I had gone without lunch and it was soon home time for the others as I heard him shout to her, "Those little bastards be home soon," next the door opened he pulled me out "get in there bitch" he shouted, I went in to the living room, she stood there with that smirk on her face, "you little bitch" she shouted, "do you think that people will believe a ugly shit like you over us," she shouted, "No" I replied, as I had obviously encountered. "What you got to say for your self?" She said as she punched me in the face, "sorry would be a start" they both shouted, I just stared at them both. Well I looked up and said "sorry," as I was afraid not to say it, "well that is not the end of it," she claimed, "now get to bed." as I walked past them Bumble kicked me.

She started laughing. I just hated her so much.

In bed I lay curled up in a ball, and I just prayed to god that he would put a stop to this abuse. Feeling so alone unhappy and cared, I really didn't want to fall asleep as I dreaded to face the next day.

I hid under my covers and that's where I stayed till morning.

That morning I got up got washed and dressed did a few of my jobs, and went down stairs to see Bumble in the kitchen, "I suppose you will want breakfast" she said, being the cocky tart she was.

I looked at her and said "Yes please" she handed me a plate with the night before dinner on "eat that" she sneered as she passed it to me and spat in it. She left the room as she did she slapped my head saying I was repulsive.

I scraped the dinner in the bin and went without. I continued with my jobs and got ready for school, I was made and example of to the others incase they tried to tell others how they came about their bruises and marks.

No one said a word to me I just got a smile from Lizzie and Roy that said enough to me.

I set off to school I got there as the bell went. I entered in to my class and sat down, I was very quiet that day, and I couldn't look at Mr Fen. He betrayed me, betrayed my trust. From that day on I hated Mr Fen and school. But I was to leave and start at the prêt school soon, I was only to glad to see the back of Mr Fen. I couldn't wait to leave. I spent the rest Of my days at that school not telling anything or trusting Mr. Fen at all.

A few days Later Mr Fen sent a letter home to my father telling him how my school work had deteriorated, as he had done many a time another reason for him to give me a belting. But no one wanted to know why my school work was under grades.

I hated my father and Bumble and Mr Fen and school. I felt so alone and unhappy, soon July came round and I left Gates Junior School, I couldn't bring my self to say goodbye to Mr. Fen.

The next few months came and went so quick, the same abuse that didn't end but my secondary school was more interesting.

I meet many new friends, and the days were happier at school.

It was during my first year that I realised others never had the life at home that I endured; expect the odd one, most were poor no one had much money but the friends I had made were happy at home and they soon got to know and understand how home life was for me.

They understood about my bruises and cuts, as some came to witness on a few accounts that both my father and Bumble lashed out at me, they became too scared to knock for me for school as Dad or Bumble was very abusive to them for knocking, soon I was to me them at the top of the road.

CHAPTER 6

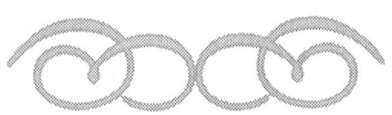

SO ALONE

As time went my thoughts were of the past, mum, my sisters and brothers, I would pray for the day I too would escape out of this hell hole, surviving this hell I wondered if I ever would.

I had visions of not living beyond sixteen. I really thought I would be murdered before then with the beatings I got or by going hungry.

Soon Lizzie started work earning her own money, so she thought, but dad and Bumble took the whole of her wages from her, leaving her with no money to get to and from work, nothing for food during the day, and she was not allowed to take a packed lunch. When Lizzie started this job dad and Bumble would show up any time of the day, Lizzie would dread this as she was made to hand over papers and what ever else they demanded, which was more so giving Lizzie a pound and she having to give them change of five pound, only out of sheer fear she did this and out of guilt as dad and Bumble would make her feel, as he they did with us all. All decisions where made for us, none of us had a say about anything, we were all too afraid to argue. With all the abuse I actually became to feel we was just there for her beck and call, a worthless nothing as she often told me.

On one occasion things got tough for Lizzie while working at that place, even more now. One day our older sisters walked into the shop were Lizzie worked, instead of rushing over to them to embrace them with kisses and hugs and tears of joy, she froze; there was nothing more she would have wanted after not being allowed to see them for years, to rush into their arms and hug and kiss them. But her response was of sheer fear and panic incase dad or Bumble came in to catch her talking to Sandy and Jane, she see the look upon Sandy and Jane's faces as they saw Lizzie's. She heard one say "let's go she doesn't know us." The pain and guilt she suffered, she had to live with. Knowing they were hurt as such as she was. Knowing she never had the chance to explain this to either of them. She was too scared to speak about this as anything else that happened. Like every one else had to bottle up their emotions, anger and fear, because of reprisals from dad and Bumble.

In which we all knew what these reprisals would entail.

None of us was allowed to have or show our feelings.

As time went by Lizzie met a lad Reg as time went they became besotted with each other, Reg found the courage to ask dad if he could marry Lizzie, to our surprise he agreed, the engagement took place at our house, a month later as Lizzie was getting ready to go out he asked her "where do you think you're going"? She replied "out with Reg" "oh no you don't you can get round there and end it now" he snapped at her. Upset and petrified and out of sheer fear she went and told Reg.

"My father has ordered me to finish the engagement and I am not allowed to see you again." Reg was mortified, but knew for Lizzie's sake not to question our father, days later dad took her to Regs house to collect her engagement presents in which he and Bumble sold those days later.

Soon after Lizzie stood up to our father and left home. Like all the others we were not allowed to mention her name. Now it was Roy's turn Roy had a little job where he earned a few bob, for our father to take this from him, he started to work all the hours he could, Roy had fallen in love with another by now Ellie. Roy's boss helped him to get a flat all behind dads back; Roy intended to leave home as soon as he turned sixteen. On the day of his sixteenth birthday, he came strutting towards the house with a fag in his mouth, not a care in the world.

Dad saw him, "You can take that out your mouth and I'll have that now" he shouted at Roy. Roy looked at him he said "You wish, you bastard. I'm sixteen now and I can do what I like" dad started to go for Roy, Roy stood his ground, he said "Ye you bloody bastard I'll knock you straight on your arse" dad looked at Roy in amazement then said "Don't you dare talk to me like that I'll knock all sorts of shit out of you" "Come on then" Roy said, "Try it you bastard, for years I've been punched and kicked by you and her, and that ended yesterday" Roy told him.

"I've took all sorts of shit from you and that evil bastard you call your tart, fuck off out my way" Roy shouted as he pushed past. I was gob smacked at the fact Roy kept his word the promise he made him self, that when he was sixteen he'd stand up to dad, and he did. With the shock of Roy standing up to him, dad shouted 'Get out get out my house you are not welcome here any more'.

"Welcome" Roy shouted back, "This is a fucking hell hole, and as for you slinging me out, I left yesterday. I've come for my stuff" he walked to go indoors, leaving dad outside gob smacked. Roy wandered in to see Bumble stood in the door way, "You are Not Welcome Here" she said all brazen, "Get out my fucking way you; you evil twisted bastard" Roy said to her.

As Roy pushed past her, she ran in the living room and shouting "ED, ED come in here quick." Not so brave then I thought.

Roy collected his few bits and headed off towards the Main rd, telling me before he left, "Sorry girl I love you, see you soon, ye I'll be back for you." I stood there, the tears just ran down my face I was all alone now. I felt empty and scared. I knew Roy would not be back, Dad wouldn't allow that.

I stood and watched Roy as he walked out of site, the tears just rolled down, I felt so sick. Soon dad was shouting out "Get in here you; ya bitch and he won't be seeing you again I'll see to that." He meant it.

I went in doors, closed the front door and was ordered to make tea, and then go clear out Roy's things he had left behind to get rid of any of his presence in the house. I made the tea took it in to them and walked up stairs, as I heard them rowing by now about Roys money, I took up a carrier bag or two to clear anything Roy had left, I sorted his room and bagged up what he had left and I took it down placed it by the back door, returned up stairs to strip his bed, I clutched his sheets in my arms that I had screwed up, sat on his bed and cried. Soon they were calling me down. I went in to see what they wanted, I just knew it wouldn't be long, "well" they said "looks like its all down to you, washing ironing the ruddy lot you can thank that pissing lot that's deserted you, so piss off and start by washing up and you can make more tea", they ordered. I headed for the kitchen in tears.

In tears I washed the dishes, cleaned the kitchen, and washed the floor returned up stairs to clean Roy's room sweep and wash the floor,

I return down stairs to make more tea as I was ordered to do. As I was washing up and dried the cups, I was told I would not be returning back to school as often, my help was needed at home. I just looked at him and her, and said nothing.

While doing my chores they were having a row, nothing unusual at that.

It then turned in to a fight; I didn't know what about I didn't care. They called me in still shouting at each other, they questioned me about something in the past I told them I didn't remember, to be told I was a liar.

I did remember it was regards to Debs and how she was treated by them, and regards to a fox fur coat that Nan our dad's mother had given Lizzie. The very day she got it dad said "Bumble wanted to borrow it for that night" as they were going out, as they often did, for Bumble to return to tell Lizzie she lost it; we all knew she sold that fur coat. But I knew that whatever I said it would be wrong and another reason for a punch or a kick. I tried to avoid getting tangled in their rows and fights.

The row got worse she threw a punch at him, pulling me on the settee as they struggled, with that she grabbed my leg and stubbed her fag out, I screamed and got free from her, I ran up stairs to the bathroom and locked my self in, the pain was unreal, the head of the fag was still stuck to my leg. As much as I cried, there was no escaping how was I to survive this abuse I wondered.

Things only got worse. Soon it went quiet I was called down. I went down entered in she told me I got what I deserved! He just laughed, "Your leg is not that bad so don't play on it" he shouted at me.

The day was mad them fighting and rowing as I tried to pass by them she stood and stared at me, the front rooms in a mess total mess, I was ordered to clean it up, there was broken cups ashtrays dog ends every where, I went and got the dust pan brush and started to clear up.

As I picked up the poker it brought back the memories to the time dad ordered Roy to go at the end of the garden to collect the wind fall of apples from next doors tree, he left a foot print in the dirt, dad went mad he called everyone out, where we all had to take a shoe off and hand it to him, he put every shoe into the print until one fitted, of course it was Roy's.

He grabbed hold of him dragging in him in doors, threw him to the floor and he laid in to him, kicking and hitting him in the stomach head and back Roy was screaming in pain begging him to stop, Bumble goading him on "go on Ed go on kick him go on," Lizzie was screaming "leave him alone leave him, he as not done anything wrong leave him" as Roy's screamed wailed over Lizzie's, Dad continued to kick and she continued to goad him on, I tried to pull dad off Roy screaming to leave him alone but she pulled my jumper pulling me away and hitting me.

I got up ran to the fire place grabbed the poker and put it across dad's back screaming at him "leave him alone." That instant he stopped, I could see the pain in his face, like I cared, but he left Roy alone, he turned to me, Lizzie ran to Roy's aid to help him, his face in blood, he could hardy move, dad stepped forward and looked at me, "you bastard" he called me, I legged it, to the front door realising he couldn't run, but I did, I knew if he caught up with me I'd be in for a beating, I opened the door as I ran she grabbed me, boy did he belt me, I couldn't sit down for a week.

But my concerns were for Roy, what dad did to Roy you would not have treated an animal the way he treated Roy, there was no need for his actions that day, like there was no reason for his actions any day, and her she goaded him that made her as bad, she enjoyed to see us cry, Roy was to receive no medical attention. Like a form of entertainment I heard them calling me again.

I put back the poker with tears in my eyes. Then I went to see what they wanted now. I was still thinking of that day with Roy.

Remembering the state of Roy's body and how later that day a neighbour knocked and asked what all the screaming was about, Dad told him we were playing he said "Sounded to me someone was being murdered."

Dad told him to piss off if he knew what was good for him, later that night Dad claimed we dreamt it.

I was surely wondering were they a pair of psychopaths that we lived with. We knew what we saw but no one dare argue with him.

With that I heard them calling louder, here I go again I say to my self little slave girl, back to reality.

I was told to fill the coal bucket, couldn't understand why, as it was a hot day but I did it. Filling it up I remember not long ago, one of the mind games he played with us all then was to take out the coal from the shed, sweep the dust and put the coal back, the mind games, and how this particular day Bumble see me covered in black coal dust dragged me up stairs and scrubbed my face with vim an sourer that we washed the bath out in, calling me a little bastard telling me I was a waste a space.

Leaving my face grazed and sore, I remember back how Jake questioned my face the next day, "What the hell" He said She looked at me as I her as much as I wanted to tell him but I knew better. "That stupid bastard washed her face in vim didn't you" She shouted. We both knew that she knew that she did it.

I bowed my head and said nothing. Jake hugged and kissed me, "you silly girl" he said, not sure if Jake believed her. Jake was seven years older than I he was so gentle, and dad and Bumble secmed scared of him, Jake was of stocky build and she never seemed to sure of Jake when he was home. To discover, Jake was scared of them as we all were, but Jake new what they was carrying on before mum died, he was Dad's cover up, used Jake to do what he was doing behind mum's back.

The tears fell as I topped the coal bucket up took it in, I was reminded of the chores to be done washing ironing cleaning the lot, nothing I wasn't doing at 8years old but then I had my siblings to help, I was so alone I missed them all so much I felt so worthless as she always told me I was, I actually started to believe I was. The curtain never moved for me.

But for me my life got harder, autumn came as my birthday approached not happy birthday nothing, but I really didn't care, it was just another day on to getting out of this hell hole. Like my last birthday just another day.

Doing the chores that day was no different from any other day I rinsed the bottles and put them out in the hall way, while I washed the floor on my hands and knees.

She came in and pushed me down as I got up she slipped on the wet floor, this was a   reason for her to tell me I was an ugly bitch and I should have died with my mother as she often would say with a punch in my face to follow. Despite all the kicks punches and physical abuse it did not hurt anymore, it were the mental things she said now that really hurt especially about my Mum!

I continued to put the bottles out in hope to see Martin as I'd seen most mornings from the window. Martin was the milk mans helper, a nice tall handsome lad, I really liked him, as I walked towards the door she'd shout "hurry up bitch with the milk," I know who you are looking out for, and why would he look at an ugly bitch like you" she'd shout at me. But I ignored her remarks.

As I brought it in putting it in the fridge she'd slap my head, "bitch" she'd say, that was all I ever got these days.

I wished I'd gone to school everyday, it was only when the school board man come I had to go for 2 to 3 days but I loved being at school to get away from them.

The next day she was moaning she was bored, and I could not help myself to say well if you got up and helped may be you wouldn't be so bored, the anger on her face was a picture, she walked towards me "you nasty little bitch" she sneered at me. I said in my defence, "I'm nasty well I wonder what that makes you bitch," I shouted back, she came hurling at me, "if I get my bleeding hands on you you're dead," she claimed, I looked at her and laughed, and walked away, leaving her to scream abuse, I ignored her and went upstairs . Hours later she grabbed my neck, "you listen here bitch don't ever talk to me like that again or I'll break your neck, you ugly little shit" she said. I pulled away and stared at her, so full of hate she spat at me, an hour later dad came in, "hey get your shoes on get up the shop" he said to me, "where did you get money from?" she asked him, "window cleaning money you nosey cow" he said. Then go to the chip shop he told me, "What we having chips then" she screamed at him. "well ye you dozy cow not unless you or her want to cook" he shouted at her.

Off I went to the chip shop and newsagents I didn't need a second telling, never had that here before ever .I had a chance to view the Christmas decorations in the shops, as even Christmas was so different when mum was alive. Christmases then were Christmases to remember.

I ran all the way, as I queued I saw one of the Taylor boys, "hi ya girl not seen you for a while how are ya?" "Don't see you at school much these days either whys that?" he asked.

I explained I have to help out at home now, "Ha the little slave girl" he said, "how about you and I going out Sunday, I know that's the day your old man lets you out," I smiled and said "no thanks, but I'd rather not" "Why got your eyes on another have you?" He said "one of Roy's friends?" "No" I replied. "Oh you know how to break some ones heart don't you?" he called out. "If I say please would you think about it?" he shouted out.

"No thanks" I shouted back. I got served and left, he waited outside "Oh go on" he said. I said "Push off your chips will get cold." He laughed and said "One day you'll regret it," I laughed and said "you wish," and set of home. I got home and she dished up the chips, being the evil cow she was she again spat in mine has she handed me the plate.

With that Dad called her, she put her plate on to the side and went to see what he wanted, and while she was gone I swapped plates, and went and sat in the diner alone and eat them, with a big smile upon my face.

The best Christmas I had in a long time, got my own back. As Christmas in this house was nothing to write home about as the saying went.

After tea I had to wash and dry up the dishes, made them a cuppa, I ran the bath for my self, I kneeled on the floor put my arms folded onto the bath and lay my head down, my thoughts went back to mum again remembering my bath times, how she'd warm the towel by the open fire, and as I got out the bath she would wrap the towel around me, and dry me so gentle, I also thought about my siblings and where they might be and what they would be doing and were they missing me as I was them. Soon I was brought back to reality, with dad calling me to hurry up. I soon bathed and got dressed and headed down stairs, the thought of the laundrette made me tired, but I had to go to the laundrette as the wash tub had broken.

As I got ready and bagged up the washing dad shouted out "leave that till tomorrow now get up to bed" I did as I was told.

Next morning after all the jobs were done I headed off to the laundrette, a nice bright febuary day, struggling with two big bags, I finally got there, as I entered in Tony Carter was there, "Blimey hello stranger" he said, "don't see you about much these days," "no" I replied "I can't be ruddy Cinderella and have a social life," he Laughed, "ah well you still got sense a humour." "So you got to do the washing for your old mum ye," I glared at him and said "She is not my ruddy mother she is my father's tart and if you repeat what I just said you'll regret it." "No I won't say anything honest" he said, then began to tell me "My parents hate your dad and his tart, they have a good idea what they do to you lot, evil gits, many do round here, but no one can prove it, ya dad is such an intimidating so and so gets away with murder". He told me. "Well my mum was in the shop the other day sees your dads tart, she told my Mum you lot was right little bastards and how she hates you all." "Really" I said "when was this then"! "Just after Christmas" he said. "Well feelings are mutual". I replied. "Well I can't blame you" he replied. He collected his washing and went on his way. "See you around then yes?" He called as he left the laundrette.

Soon my washing was done I bagged it up and set off home, struggling to carry it, I finally made it home. As I got in I left the washing by the back door, to hear "that you?" Put the kettle on wash them few dishes up before you hang that lot out, I made the tea and washed the few dishes in the sink, and continued to sort the washing out and hang it on the line, I was so fed up with the way life was I burst in to tears, I picked up the empty basket and went inside. To hear her call my name and say "make some more the tea," I ignored her I was tired and not feeling too well and I felt very down, fed up being the slave girl. She came running at me "did you hear me? You lazy bitch" she shouted, she became abusive again mentally and physically. "It's your bloody fault she screamed at me." I couldn't be bothered to ask what. I ran inside and I locked my self in the bathroom nursing my wounds mentally and physically and stayed there till she calmed down.

Dad did various jobs these days away from the house she spent most of her time up the town gambling ,on many occasions she came back with the hump and I had to go looking for dad, other days he came home with the hump and I had to go looking for her up the town.

On one occasion she came home moaned and swore, I had to run round looking for him there was his ladder propped against the wall in Goodman's way but no him.

I called and called, but got no answer I see his bucket, but not him. So I knocked, called out in the house where the ladders were. I heard voices I wasn't sure so I pushed open the front door and there he was in the arms of another women.

I ran, he came out running after me shouting "wait". But I ran home. I told her that he was coming.

Over the next few days he mellowed. By the 3rd day he caught up with me in the kitchen. Bumble was in bed. He mentioned making a cuppa tea.

"You alright girl?" he asked, I glared at him, "tea you telling me to make it, or offering" I replied, "no I'll make it" he said.

It was then I realised I had a hold over him.

I turned to him and said "You're making me a cuppa a tea," "ye if you go get the milk in" he replied. Off I went to front door and opened it, to see the milk float pulling away, "damn"

I said, "Missed him," I picked up the milk and headed for the kitchen, "there you go two pints of milk" I said. "Oh ye right" he replied, as he poured the milk in to the tea he turned to me and said "about the other day you won't mention about me will you?" I stared at him "mention what? Telling her about you and your girl friend in your arms?" I said, "ye that" he replied. He passed my tea and said "well"? With that Bumble came in and shouted at me "where is my bloody tea"? She went to hit me. "Don't hit her, dad told her, I made the tea," "YOU?" she said.

I realised he was running scared. I looked at her and grinned. "You bitch" she shouted, dad shouted at her "oi no need for that." That was the first time ever he stuck up or me, but for his own reasons of course. She stormed out. I need a pair Shoes I told him.

"A fiver enough?" he said. "Yes, good fine" I replied as he put his hand in his pocket, and handed me a fiver. "You can go out with your mates if you like" he snapped. "Well yes I will" I sneered. "Leave the chores today" he said. Well I thought, he is worried in case she finds out. I finished my tea put the cup in the sink and headed up stairs to get ready. Twenty minutes and I was gone out the door up the road. Shouting "FREEDOM" as a man approached me, "your old man in" he said, "knock and find out" I said, and went on. Thinking no more about it, Off I went to the shoe shop, spent ages choosing a pair. Finally settling for a pair of dolly shoes I went to my friend Sue's house. Her mum answered "hello come on in, err" she said "is that true about your dad having a fling with Mrs G." "I don't know" I said, "well the whole streets talking about it, and there was a terrible to do there last night" she claimed. I shrugged my shoulders and never commented. "Sue in" I said, "No she's gone on a few errands for me, waits for her if you like she shouldn't be too long now" said Mrs Cooper. "No thank you I'll call back later for her" I said, "ok girl" she said as I left.

I made my way to Sandy's house. I ran up to the bus stop and got a bus to town, as I had some change left from the shoe money. She didn't know I was coming so I only hoped she'd be in, or even still lived there. I got off at the top of her road, excited but nervous would she remember me? I wondered. I walked down the street stopping outside where I lived when mum was alive, and cried, so many lovely memories to recall at that house with mum, I thought, and walked slowly around the corner, there it was as I had remembered. I walked up the path hesitating to knock, I stood there for a moment, and I thought well I've come this far and knocked, no one answered I waited, then the door opened my brother in law stood there "Bloody hell" he said "Jess that you"? "come on in" he said as he gave me a big hug," "haven't you grown he said" shouting out "SANDY look who's here what a surprise," I followed him up the hall, he open the kitchen door, "look who's here" he said to her as she stood frozen on the spot.

Sandy looked hard, "oh my god" she cried. Hugging me, "After all these years, you remembered where we lived." She cried, I cried as we hugged, "Oh! I don't believe this" she kept saying "you were only seven when I last saw you" she said and cried. Allen made a cup of tea, while Sandy and I chatted away. She got out all the photos and we looked for ages. "Jane would love to see you too," after we had tea we walked to Jane's it was not too far away, she was pleased to see me as I her, we all hugged and kissed. It was an emotional time. I discovered I'd got two nieces and a nephew from Sandy and Allen. I remembered Allen junior but he was only six months old last time I saw him it was near to eight years on now. I also had a niece from Jane. What a lovely day it was, but I had to get back now as it was approaching 5pm. I said my goodbyes and promised I'd see them again soon.

I headed home back on the bus, going over the day, and how lovely it was to see them again after so long. But knew it had to be kept secret. Soon the bus was at my stop. I got off and walked home, still on cloud nine, as I turned into my turning I wondered what was in store as I got in. I approached the gate way to hear shouting, here we go again I thought, knocked at the door, dad answered and told me Mrs P has been knocking for you" he shouted at me, "ok" I said, heading for the kitchen. Next Bumble came out the living room shouting "where the hell you been all day?" I looked at her and replied "Out." "Well you didn't do any bloody chores did you? You bitch." She continued to shout. With that dad come in, "Mrs P has been here I don't know how many times she wants her dog took out! Get over there and do that" he said. I turned around to the front door and headed to Mrs P's. I knocked loudly, shouting "it's only me" Mrs P came to the door, "hello dear come on in". She said.

"I've been over to yours, I don't know how many times today" she said, "Yes I was told you want the dog took out" I said, "No I just said that to get you over here" she chuckled," "Oh right" I replied. "What's up then?" I said. "Well I've been chatting to my sister, the one that works up the school, as a dinner lady" she said "and she was telling me about Bumble, how she knows her from the past" "oh yes" I said "Well I think Bumble has cottoned on to who my sister and I are, so be careful Incase she asks you anything" she said. I looked at her, "and"? I said.

"Oh yes the cuts and bruises you poor girl, yes we know all about your father and that tart he is with, and giving away their own child", she explained to me "so keep it to your self for now my dear" she said. "We'll chat later", she said. Surprised as I was she knew so much I headed off home. As I was about to cross the road I saw Jim the milkman "hello girl" he shouted "you ok? An't seen you smile in ages," he said. "Seen Martin yet" he shouted, I knew what he meant; he had seen me looking out the window to catch a glimpse of Martin. "You you'll get there" he said, Sure we will Jim I called back.

I got indoors to be interrogated, "What did she want? What did she say?" they said, I told them she already took the dog out as it got late. "LIAR" she shouted at me and smacked me around the ear. Now what did she say, "nothing" I said. "You know better not to tell Mrs P anything", she said to me and you won't be going over there again" Bumble told me. I just stared at her and went up stairs. Dad came up "get your shoes did you?" He said "and how was Sandy and that lot?" he shouted at me, I was shocked to hear what he had just said, and stared at him. "What" I said, "Oh don't give me all that you lying bitch you think I'm stupid don't you?" As he hit me around the face, He shouted as he punched me in the chest with that evil look in his eye and that look upon his face. "You ever go behind my back again god help ya" he told me.

"Oh and don't worry about the other day that was sorted earlier and you owe me a fiver" he said as he left my room. Then I realised what Sue's mum was on about. But still wondered how he knew I had gone to see Sandy.

I lay on my bed holding my chest that was giving me a lot of pain from him punching me. I wondered when it was all going to end. I just lay and cried, as I lay on my bed my thoughts went back to my brothers and sisters and the day. Wishing I could curl up and die, to escape this abusive life of mine.

I cried my self to sleep.

Chapter 7

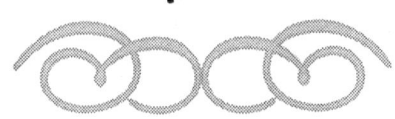

Come what may

The next morning I got up I heard the sounds of the milk bottles I went out to take the milk in, there was Martin, I stood and chatted to him for a few minutes, he told me his address and walked away smiling, Dad came into the kitchen, he grabbed my arm and said "you ever go behind my back again I'll knock all sorts of shit out you do you hear me?" "Yes dad" I replied.

I knew he was referring to going to see my sister behind his back. Still not sure how he knew I went I'll never know as I told no one. But I wasn't to concern about that right now I had Martin on my mind.

Days went by I still had Martin on my mind, what had I to loose, I plucked up the courage to ask could I go out tomorrow.

He looked at me and said "I'll see if your chores are done." I walked away and said nothing. Next day came I got up even earlier to do all my chores shattered as I was I sat down for a moment, staring at the curtains that stayed open day in day out. The curtains never moved, and nor did my life. I got back up and carried on; I heard movement from up stairs. They were getting up I went and put the kettle on as I knew that would be my next job. The food still under lock and key and anything in the fridge was marked up, I couldn't have breakfast.

I made the tea as dad and Bumble came in the kitchen. I handed them their tea, then went up to make their bed and tidy up, as I made dad and Bumbles bed I noticed a letter under her pillow addressed to her, I just looked at it and put the pillow back and left the room, as I got out side she came charging up the stairs pushing me back into their room, screaming at me, you've read my bloody letter, as she grabbed me by my hair pulling me to the floor and kicking me, as she screamed for dad to come up, "ED ED Get up here" he came charging up the stairs "what's going on?" he said. "Her she's read my letter" waving it in the air by now, "bitch you bitches," she screamed. I managed to get up dad told her to go downstairs she did, he looked at me and laughed and headed down stairs him self. I just knew that was it there was no chance of going out now, I went into the bathroom to wash and tend my wounds, then went down.

As I was about to enter the living room they started to row. The row turned into a fight, I went and stayed in the kitchen, after a while she came out and stormed upstairs, dad called me in, I went in to see what he wanted, "Did you read that letter?" he asked I said "no dad" as I was looking at the state of the room I'd cleaned not so long ago.

In a toned voice, I said "I'm sure, I see it covered it and left the room" "ok" he said "you better be telling me the truth go on get out to the kitchen" he said, so I turned and went, he soon followed me, Bumble came down, in tears, "you'd better get in there an clean that mess up" he ordered me, raising my eyebrows I went in to do it, there was all torn up photos over the place torn too small to see who they were of.

I cleared up the mess and put the cushions back, and went back to the kitchen, they went back in the living room, next thing dad called me, "were going out, you can piss off out and be back here by 7pm" he said. I couldn't believe what I was hearing, I ran up stairs had a wash down got dressed got my 2s 6d I had hid and went out, I ran up the road despite my back arm and leg hurting. I couldn't go to Martins yet it was too early, so I went over to the cemetery again and sat beside mum's grave side. Telling her how much I missed her, I found it very comforting to sit there I felt reassured for some reason, after an hour I headed for Martins, up to the Main rd, I went on to Martins as I got to his street I pondered to go and knock at his door, my heart pounding, but I did I walked up the path and knocked, Martins dad answered the door, "hello I'm sorry to trouble you but is Martin in please" I said " No not yet but he shouldn't be too long come in and wait for him" he said.

I followed him into the living room where Martins mum sat on the sofa with his two little sisters, "What's your name?" they asked me as I was about to answer Martin came in he saw me sat there and the smile on his face said it all,

"Hello" he said, "Hello" I replied, "Fancy going for a walk" he said "love to" I replied, as we set off out. We got to the end of his street and he held my hand. "Where shall we go?" he asked "don't mind" I replied.

We walked hand in hand and ended up at the local park, we sat and watched the swans on the pond, and chatted a while about anything and everything. After a while we just sat quiet we were just glad to be with each other Martin put his arm around me and held my hand. It was a nice sunny day but a little chilly as being February. The day went by too quick and soon I had to return home, Martin walked me home where on our way we made arrangements to see each other the next day.

We soon reached my house, we stood out side hid by the bushes, Martin had his arms around me holding me, as we kissed and said goodnight I saw my father watching us from an upstairs window, As Martin and I parted for the night and I went in.

There dad stood with a smirk on his face, "Have fun did you" he said. I looked at him and said "yes thank you", I went into the kitchen made a cup of tea and looked to see if there was anything to eat, but there was nothing, so I headed for the living room, I sat down, and Bumble just stared at me I could see she had been crying.

But I said nothing I just sat and drank my tea. Dad entered in and she shouted at him, "you going to tell her then? Or should I?"

In temper he shouted back at her "just leave it shut up for Christ sake." I just looked away feeling uncomfortable. I asked would it be alright if I went to bed. Dad looked at me and said "suppose so." I got up from where I was sitting and quickly walked out of the room.

I headed up stairs as quick as my legs would carry me. I gathered my nightdress and headed for the bathroom. I got washed and dressed for bed and headed back to my room.

I lay on my bed and wondered if Martin had got back home alright, and thought about the lovely day I had had, excited and butterflies in my tummy just thinking of Martin.

To feel safe, happy and wanted, with Martin, for someone to care about me for me, this was a wonderful feeling.

As I lay there I could hear raised voices, they had started to argue again, as they did I wondered what it was she wanted dad to tell me. As much as I wanted to know I daren't ask, but it did puzzle me now to know what it was all about.

Soon it went quiet and dad came up to my room, get up get dressed run up the off-licence and get me 10 fags, and don't take too long. As quick as I could I got dressed collected the money and made off to the off-licence and back again as I entered in the front door which I left on ajar I could hear them shouting at each other, I knocked on the living room door and waited, "what?"

Dad called out, "your fags are here" I shouted. Take them in the kitchen and make some tea I'll be out soon. I did as I was told as I finished making the tea dad came in to the kitchen, I handed him his tea and fags.

He glared at me; I just looked at him saying nothing. Next thing she shouted "you bastard I hate you, you're to blame for all this, my Life's in turmoil and all I've done is, sort out your fucking kids and be a mother to them, I left mine and I can't even see them. Now look at the mess I'm in?" she screamed. I looked at dad his face like thunder he literately slung his tea in the sink and went storming in pushing past me, shouting back at her "you fucking what you ungrateful bitch that was you're own choice you chose to leave them, and the last kid you couldn't be too sure who's she was, one minute she was mine and when it suited you she was his you were no fucking mother, you gave her up to him I never fucking asked you to do that" by now she started screaming and attacking him like a possessed woman and shouting back "I told you she was yours long ago you bastard, you know why we both decided to give her up."

I presumed they were talking about Debs.

Next thing I heard things being smashed, And her screaming "I hate you I hate you And I hated your fucking kids all of them."

As I stood in the kitchen listening I was amazed the whole street didn't hear all this, as for her hating us well we knew that, and feelings were mutual, and as for her being a mother well I thought that's an understatement. She wouldn't know what the word mother meant.

Then Dad shouted at her "well you've torn the letter up now what's done is done and I'm sick of you keep bringing it up, fuck off back to him and your fucking kids if it keeps you happy, instead of going over old ground all the time this was years ago so why keep bringing it up for Christ sake."

She shouted back. "I wanted to see my kids and he won't let me as you read in that letter" "well come on" he shouted "you left it a bit late to decide" next it went quiet, then, expect for the sounds of her echoes with crying. Dad came out to the kitchen "put the kettle on and make it sharp" he said to me.

Grinning away I said "Yes dad" as once again like the little slave girl I made the tea. as I was pouring the tea he came back in "make hers sweet" he told me, and left. "Ok" I said as I added 4 sugars to her cup, being as she only took none or half a spoon of sugar. Then as I stirred it I spat in it and took it in "Your tea" I said. As they were now cuddling up to each other I placed it on the table.

With a big grin I left the room collected my cup of tea from the kitchen and went up to bed.

As shattered as I was I couldn't sleep, the thoughts of the argument went around in my head, well I thought maybe that's what Mrs. P was on about, and was this what she wanted dad to tell me weeks before, not that I could see that was anything I was interested in, all I could see from that argument was she did her kids a big favour at least they had a better life than any of my siblings or I did.

I then cast my mind back to Martin and drifted off to sleep.

Soon it was April, the weather was lovely my home life didn't changed much in the way of the mental or physical abuse, still the little slave girl.

But my days were to look forward to spending my time with Martin.

He kept me alive when I felt so alone and so unhappy at home.

He always made he laugh and he had a lovely sense of humour.

This particular day Martin asked if I'd like to go out to the pictures "of course I'd love to" I replied. We became very close by now Martin and me.

"Well what would you like to see?" he asked I replied "I don't mind I'll leave it to you." So we planned that Saturday coming we would go to the pictures.

Excited as I was I daren't let my feelings of how I felt bout Martin show at home, as hard as it was I had to carry on as a normal day.

Sitting down to tea that night half a plate of broken biscuits, the rows erupted again between dad and Bumble.

Nothing strange about that, I was called in to the living room and questioned about the shopping money she accused me of short changing them she had a pad and pencil in her hand.

So I had to go through everything, she passed it to me.

I stated "you gave me 10s 6d.

Bread is 1s 3d.

Spam is 9d for half a lb.

Spuds were 6d for 2lb.

10 fags are 11d

Jar of jam is 11d

Which came to 5s 4d?

Leaving you 5s 2d.

There's a 2 shilling coin for the meter in your change and the rest, 3 one shilling   coins and the odd 2d." I told them.

I added it up for them 5s 4d

5s 2d

10s 6d

She punched me in the face and shouted "Don't bloody patronise me you bitch".

Dad told me to go and clear up, as he screwed up the paper that I had written on.

Then they argued again.

Obviously over spent I told my self nothing new.

Next day he told me he had some jobs for me to do running errands for neighbours as he needed the money, strangely Mrs P was one of them, I went neighbour to neighbour on the list, there were five of them in all on my list.

Each paid me a little, together I earned 5s 6d. As usual Mrs P was so pleased to see me she kept some money by for me to save as she used to.

I returned home with money in hand and he took it.

May was Martins birthday and I was telling Mrs P She said "what ever jobs you do I'll be very grateful for and I'll help you save" I was so pleased. I hugged her.

Well Saturday came I asked dad could I go out if all my jobs were done.

He stared at me "I suppose but don't make a habit of it", he said, I went about tidying the bedrooms sweeping and washing floors, cleaned the bathroom and the toilet. Fed the dog took it out, did the errands for the neighbours by now I was absolutely shattered.   To return home intending to have a bath and get dressed ready to go out.

But Bumble found me another job to do. I had to do the Ironing which was meant to be done Sunday.

I got the table ready when dad came in, "what you are doing?" he said.

I replied "The ironing as I've been told to do."

"No leave that go out" he said. "Be in by 10-30pm" he said.

So I did no more than to get bathed and changed.

Off I went up the road to meet Martin.

As I headed up the street he was coming to meet me. Hand in hand we went off to get the bus to town to the pictures.

I was happy. All day I had thought of this moment. Just Martin and me.

We reached the stop we needed, and walked a short way to the Odeon.

Martin paid for the tickets and we headed for the screen.

We found a seat and sat ready for the film to start, the film was called The Last Grenade. I was so shattered I ended up falling asleep.

Next thing I knew it was the interval.

Martin went and got some drinks and returned.

He held my hand and I fell asleep again.

Next Martin was waking me the film had ended. I felt so guilty, but sure he would understand, holding hands.

We got the bus back and Martin walked me home.

Saying goodnight not wanting our night to end, we arranged to see each other the next day. We hugged and kissed and Martin went on his way.

As I got in it was quiet, only the hall light on.

I got to the top of the stairs, when dad appeared. Tomorrow you've got extra jobs to do he said and returned to his room, I never answered him; I just retired to my room.

Next morning soon came round there seemed to be a lot of activity going on when I got up, the cupboards were emptied out under the stairs, and the coat and shoe cupboard emptied with its contents all over the hallway floor. As I see this I took that these were the extra jobs he spoke of the night before.

I stepped over everything that lay on the floor to reach the kitchen.

Dad was in there pouring tea out. I looked at him and thought that's a first.

"I suppose you want one?" he said "yes please" I replied "well you can make your own I'm not your bloody servant" he snapped.

As I looked at him and under my breath I said "no but I suppose I'm yours." As I then reached for a cup.

As I poured my tea I said "the stair cupboards are they the extra jobs you want me to do?"

"No" he snapped "did I say they were?"

I just said "no dad" I could tell he was in a mood.

Obviously he got out the wrong side of the bed, I thought to my self.

I drank my tea as I went to walk out the kitchen he said "where you think you're going?"

I replied "to get washed and dressed".

"When you've sorted that lot out in the hall way and not before, get it tidied and put it back under" he ordered.

I thought I just asked were they the extra jobs he had said "no" basically the mind games again I thought just do it girl.

I started to sort out the items over the floor when Bumble came down slapping me round the head she said "you had better do it bloody Prompt." I said nothing just carried on.

Soon it was all done under the stairs nice and tidy with boxes of junk, they hoarded the coat and shoe cupboard now tidy, and all the rubbish and mud from the shoes all swept up, the bit of floor washed.

I returned to the kitchen to tell him I had done the jobs.

He went to check, "right you can go get washed and dressed now he ordered.

Up I went, on my return I noticed they were not talking, this made a change from the rows I thought.

I went to wash up she shoved me out the way of the sink, "piss off you" she said, "no one told you to do that yet," as she banged and cluttered the cups on the side.

No matter what I did the rest of that day she picked on me, swearing slapping me around the head, or just being nasty in general, by the things she said.

I went to dad and said "no matter what I try to do job wise she's having ago at me so what do I do now?"

"Do you room and piss off out." He said.

Be back here by 8pm ish.

Dad and she seemed to avoid each other.

The morning was strange she spent most of her time in the kitchen or in and out the garden not really doing anything just slating me off if not me dad.

I didn't know what had gone on for them to be as they were this day, but deep down I really didn't care. I got the broom and pan and brush and went to do my room. Soon it was all done, not a lot had to be done really as I kept my room tidy all the time.

I got my self sorted and went to meet Martin.

I was a little quiet that day and a few times he asked "are you alright?" I just replied "yes thank you" I so much wanted to tell him what was going on but I daren't.

Incase dad questioned me.

I just wanted to be alone with Martin that day so we walked and sat in the park, which I liked to do, just him and me, we sat there for hours just talking about music, and the latest films out.

The time seemed to go too quick before I realised it was 6pm ish, so I thought it best to head home and see what lies ahead there.

But I had had a nice day with Martin, I felt now I could face what may lie ahead at home. Martin always made me laugh I just loved his sense of humour. He was so kind, and caring. He kept me in spirit.

Martin walked me home as we said good night, we arranged to meet not the next day but the day after as Martin had a few things to do. I hated the days away from Martin the time couldn't go quick enough to see him again.

I entered in to peace and quite. They were still avoiding each other, no dinner was cooked again, I hadn't got in the door 5 minutes dad called, "run to the shop get me 10 fags" he said off I went to the shops, thought I might catch up with Martin but there was no sign of him.

I got the fags and returned home. No thank you no nothing. By now she was in the living room, dad pondered in and out the garden slamming the door as he did so.

On the side was some bread I made my self a jam sandwich.

I washed up and mopped the kitchen floor.

By 9 o'clock I was shattered, I made a cup of tea and went to my room.

By now I heard doors slamming; I just ignored this and read a book.

Soon I drifted off to sleep.

Next I was being woken up, I looked at my clock, it said 12 midnight, I looked up to see Bumble "get up and go follow your father his going to kill himself." I was a bit dazed I got up, "move it" she screamed at me.

I got up got dressed as quick as I could.

Down the stairs out the door, towards the Main road. looking right and left to see if I could see dad. There he was to the right just catching a glimpse as we got to the top of the hill.

I ran after him shouting "dad wait up."

He continued to walk; I finally caught up with him.

"I suppose she sent you didn't she?" he snapped at me.

"Yes" I said. "That bloody tart he said "she's one ungrateful bitch, soon as I'm out of her way the better" he snapped.

"Where are you going dad?" I asked.

"Where I'm going is I'm going to jump off the bloody railway bridge and end it all." He said not sure how to feel about this situation I said "Dad there are no more trains till morning" "oh piss off" he said.

"Piss off and leave me alone."

"I can't can I"? I said.

"She makes me sick she's ungrateful nothing makes her happy, so what's the bloody point" he said.

As by now he was climbing up on to the bridge. "Piss off leave me alone" he kept saying.

"Dad I shouted get down you're making a fool of your self, there are no trains till morning" "Piss off" he said.

"I am determined to do my self in" he shouted at me.

I shouted back "There's the rivers up there jump in that."

I turned to walk away.

Then dad started to shout "Where you going?"

"Home" I shouted back.

As I turned I saw him stood there on the bridge.

I continued to walk away.

Next thing he was shouting "wait you bitch."

As I turned again I saw him getting down from the bridge.

I walked fast and then started to run towards home. I couldn't handle this.

As I turned to see where he was I saw him running behind me.

"Wait" he shouted. So I stopped in my tracks.

He soon caught up with me.

"I'll came back later" he said "when the trains are running."

I just looked at him, and nodded my head in disbelief.

All these bloody mind games again. That's what all this was about I thought to myself.

I felt sick and shaky. Longing for my bed now as I was really shattered.

Soon we returned home, I just headed for my bed, where I lay and felt sick and so shook up with what had gone on. I burst into tears.

Could I really handle much more here I thought.

I felt I was cracking up.

I couldn't sleep at all I felt so churned up.

I lay there and put my thoughts to Martin, I thought about the day we just had together and felt a little better.

My thoughts went back to my siblings too, wondering what they would be doing these days.

But I concentrated my thoughts on Martin.

Thinking of the hours we had to spend apart.

Soon the morning was here.

Tired as I was I got up to face the day.

As I went down stairs, I saw dad had slept in the chair and Bumble on the settee.

I really didn't feel too good. I made the tea, and sat at the back door for a little fresh air.

Thinking about the early hours I really didn't have any sympathy for him.

I just felt I had, had enough of the life I endured here. When was it all going to end?

The curtains never moved. This was a true collection of how my life, as that never moved either in this house.

The day seemed weird, when they got up they were like a couple of love birds, kissing and hugging, this was all too much for me.

Ordered to make them tea and toast, I did with little effort in it.

Dad came in the kitchen.

We're off out today you can get on with your jobs while we're out. He told me.

I finished doing the tea and toast, and took this in to them where they sat hand in hand.

Before long they had got ready and gone out. I started up stairs and worked down, making beds sweeping and washing floors, I cleaned the stairs and continued to clean down stairs, the living room diner and kitchen. Feeling tired and very tearful I started to do the washing, up to my arm pits in dirty clothes, I sorted them out in piles, and began to wash them, while filling the sink with water rinsing them through the mangle in the basket out on the line.

I did 5 loads, of clothes and bedding, by now I was feeling faint with hunger.

There was nothing in the larder just a load of junk as this was now a storage area, the food still under lock and key in the diner, when there was food in the house that's were it was stored. I looked in the fridge to see a little piece of cheese and half a tomato, and on the side two slices of bread left from earlier, I made myself a cheese and tomato sandwich a cup of tea and sat on the door step to eat it, for some reason it made me think back to few year back when she spent all the money in the betting shop gambling or on their fags. There was rarely then no money for food, so I and my siblings had to walk along the sewer to pick rhubarb and every Saturday go up the market at closing time to pick up all the spec vegetables and fruit, and how degrading this was for us, but this was a way to survive to eat, otherwise we would go without food, even though the food we collected was only fit for the pigs, but it was food.

My next job was to peel some spuds; some times I didn't know why I bothered as these days' dinners were few and far. The spuds we had dad had stolen them from someone's allotment, but I had to peel some or I would get in trouble.

The day passed with me getting in and out the washing and ironing what I could, the day soon went. It was coming up to 6-30pm they were still not home. I was hungry, I thought about cooking myself some chips but if I was caught I'd have been in big trouble for that, and I tried hard not to get in their way to stop me seeing Martin. So I went hungry.

The place tidy and all the washing done and most of the ironing, I went up to my room and read a book, soon they were back.

As they entered in I was called "where are you?" dad Shouted "up here" I called back "Then get down here and make a cup of tea" he shouted.

As I went down he punched me in the chest "you fucking lazy cow" he said, I looked at him in horror "what?" I said 'I've gone through the entire house done all the washing and most of the ironing" I said to him.

"And" he replied "you haven't put the ruddy ironing away you lazy fucker" He said as he started hitting me again, I couldn't believe what I was hearing. Me! I was lazy.

I gathered up the ironing and took it up stairs and placed it on my bed ready to sort out in piles to who was whose ironing.

I returned down stairs to finish the tea.

As I took theirs in I said "I've done the potatoes."

"And" she replied "we've eaten out."

I said nothing just returned upstairs to sort the ironing.

Not long after he called me to go to the shops to get him 10 fags, I went into my room to my drawer and got 1s out, hid it in my shoe as I went down collected the fag money and ran to the shops, while I was there I got some chips from the chippie, I was so hungry. When I got back I handed him his fags.

"You had chips?" he asked, I lied and said "no" "well I can smell chips" he said.

He left it at that and I returned to finish sorting the ironing.

By the time I went down stairs Bumble was throwing up in the toilet too. Dad came in to the living room were I was tidying up, I thought sod it what had I to lose, I asked "Can I go out later please?" he looked at me "only if all your jobs are done" he said.

I walked out with a grin on my face.

After I done my jobs here I went over to Mrs P. I went to the shop to get her paper, here you go girl 2s 10d you've earned that over the weeks she smiled as she gave me the money.

"Oh brilliant" I said "I didn't know I'd earn that much" "oh believe me you have dear, and here's 6d give that to your father" she chuckled I said "thank you" and headed home.

I now had money for Martins birthday card and present I took it up and hide it in a tin in the bottom of my wardrobe under some old clothes.

I met Martin that night, he asked me "where do you want to go" I just said "for a walk-about" so much stress at home I thought but daren't say, we had a lovely evening just being together I was happy just to be with him. I felt alive and not alone. He was so kind and caring, he would hold my hand and I felt secure. I just wanted to alone with him.

I knew he was football mad so I knew what to get him for his birthday, a signed photograph of his favourite team.

The night was good as always, and days to his birthday; well he walked me home as usual. We said goodnight looking forward to the next day, as I went in dad was there.

"I've been watching you two"he said.

I never said a word, just thought yes like you used to Lizzie you pervert. I just retired to my room saying nothing to him.

Chapter 8

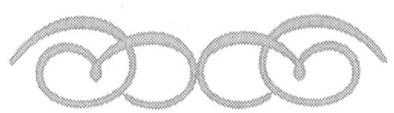

LIGHT AT THE END OF THE TUNNEL

*T*he next day I decided to go and get Martins birthday card and present, all excited I went to my wardrobe to get my tin of money.

Put it in my purse and headed up town. I brought a lovely card and the lovely football photo in a frame all wrapped nice I took it home and put it in my drawer where I thought it would be safe.

A few days later it was Martins birthday I went to my drawer got it out, took it down stairs to find a carrier to put it in. Bumble picked it up" what's this?" she asked.

I told her "Martins card and present."

"Oh really" she said "a present for lover boy" with that she got it out the wrapper.

"Leave it alone" I shouted at her.

"Leave it alone" "make me" she said, as she threw it on the floor and stamped on it I heard the glass break.

I shouted at her "You've ruined it now."

"So bloody what" she said, laughing.

As she grabbed the card and tore it up, I burst into tears, she laughed all the more.

I ran up stairs and cried more, what am I going to do now? I thought I had no way of getting any money for another few weeks.

I ran down stairs to see if I had any loose change in my pocket I found nothing.

I went and washed my face and met Martin I could only wish him happy birthday and say a card was to follow.

I felt too ashamed to tell him what had happened. He never said anything, except thank you for saying happy birthday. A few days later I earned 7d so I brought Martin the only card I could find appropriate. And gave it to him with belated in it, as the weeks went I was determine to save for another football photo for him. May be then explain why he never got a card and present on the day, not that Martin would have minded but I did.

A few days later as I asked was it alright to go out as I had done all the house work and washing, Dad agreed but paused, "Is Martin calling here to meet you" he asked "yes dad" I replied "outside" "well I want a chat with him before you two go any where" he said. I could have died, what would he want to ask Martin I thought, well the time came Martin would soon be here I ran up stairs to get bathed and changed, as I was getting ready I noticed Martin was at the gate, I ran down opened the door, "hello" he said with a big smile on his face, "you ready?" "Well not quite" I said "my dad wants to talk to you" Martin said "What's he want to talk to me about?"

"I have no idea" I said "but come in."

Martin came in, and I showed him to the living room, I introduced Martin to dad and dad to Martin, Martin sat on the settee I on the chair, dad didn't waste any time he asked Martin How much he earned and if he had he any savings,what were his intentions of work? I couldn't believe what he was asking Martin I felt so embarrassed I shut off to the conversation. I could have died with embarrassment.

I could have died there standing at the back of the settee was Bumble I was praying she wouldn't kick off; and show me up as she was keen to do, soon after an hour we were free to go.

I couldn't wait to get out of that house, so bloody money orientated he had to ask Martin things that were none of his business, I felt so ashamed.

Martin said I was a bit distant, well I had to say "nosey sod you should have told him to mind his own."

As Martin and I walked along the street I recalled he did the same to Lizzie and her boyfriend a few years back.

That's all he was interested in Money.

Well I did not let that spoil our night, Martin and I walked to the park where I liked to go so peaceful and just be with him away from others.

Martin used to say there are other places to go but I enjoyed sitting in the park.

Just talking being together was all I cared about. Martin kept me high in spirit when I was low, he taught he to believe in my self by things we talked about, and he gave me back my self esteem. I actually started to believe in myself, without

Martin I think I would have curled up in a corner and withered away.

Soon another night was near to an end, Martin and I didn't want to part but we had the next day to be together we arranged for me to meet him at his. So we headed back to my house where Martin would see me home and we both looked forward to the next day.

We said goodnight but I found it hard to leave Martin, I wanted to stay with him, he held my hand and hugged me we both said, "couldn't wait for tomorrow", we kissed and Martin headed for home. As I entered in dad stood there, I didn't say a word to him just ashamed he was my father. I went up to bed, feeling a bit sickly my self just being back home. I retired to my room.

I just lay there on my bed, wondering when all this was going to come to an end.

I looked forward to the morning to catch a glance of Martin from the window.

As the night went I was in thoughts of Martin and Dad questioning him as he did, soon I felt rough, sickly again, as I sat up on my bed I had the sudden need to rush to the toilet, just in time as I spewed up. Feeling hot and cold I didn't feel too well.

Most of that night, I was backwards and forwards to the toilet being sick.

As morning approached I heard Bumble, she must have got up early, she came up stairs and saw me being sick, with that she screamed "Oh that's bloody great Ed Ed get up here" as she pulled me by the hair.

"I bet she's Pregnant by that Martin she's being sick." I tried to tell them I wasn't pregnant I had the tummy bug that she had had, but dad pulled me out the toilet, hitting me and punching me "you stupid bitch" he screamed at me.

I fell to the floor he stamped on my leg repeatedly, swearing at me, her goading him on, I tried to get up but she kicked me in the stomach I was crying "leave me alone."

"Leave you alone" dad shouted as he punched me in the face, catching my eye.

He started to back off, I started to get up, she screamed at me allsorts I wasn't listening to her, I managed to get to the out side of my room my leg really in pain, dad shouted "you fucking stupid bitch" I shouted back "I hate you bastard" with that he punched me again and caught my other eye, he shouted "god help you if you are pregnant" I screamed through the sobs "I am not pregnant but maybe I should have been pregnant to get out this hell hole" he came rushing forward at me pushing me into my room, shouting calling me a bastard.

All the time her goading him on "Go on Ed."

As I fell on my bed he walked away shouting "you can stay in there till I tell you to come out" and went down stairs.

I lay and cried in pain my leg hurt to move it, it was swelling slightly, my stomach hurt, reaching for my bin to be sick in. My eyes red and grazed, my lip split, as I pulled my night dress up to look at my leg there was bruising up the front and back of my leg and an imprint of his boot, red and bruised on my stomach, I pulled down my night dress and looked at my ear that was red and bruised. They must really hate me I thought by now. Soon dad and Bumble shouted up they was going out.

I tried to get down stairs but as I put pressure on my leg the pain just shot up and down my leg. So I managed to get down on my bottom.

I managed to get a glass of water and found some painkillers of dads on top the fridge.

I took a few of them, and went back up stairs the way I came down, I just lay on my bed and cried.

I thought about Martin how could I get word to him, soon they came back in I could hear them laughing aloud.

I had to wait till they went to bed or go out before I could get a drink, the sickness eased as the day went by which I was glad about.

I was now concerned about Martin what would think if I didn't turn up.

Next morning I saw him and tried to get his attention, I dare not bang on the window, he left the milk and off he went. I wondered what he must have been thinking I asked myself. He wouldn't knock as he knew how dad would react, that's why I had to meet him outside in the past. Dad was like that to us all. People only came in when dad demanded.

The days went by, my leg was still in pain when I put pressure on it, one of my eyes and the bruises on my stomach were near black as the coal. Soon nearly three weeks went passed.

I heard people knock at the door, and heard dad being abusive to them telling them to piss off and not knock again, I wondered was this martin.

I returned to my room and cried.

Soon be to be called down, and told I had house work and washing to catch up on.

Still in some pain with my leg, my bruises that were now a yellow colour I stood there and looked at them remembering what Martin had said about believing and standing up for what you believe in.

I went back at them, "I'm not well enough to do housework and it's your fault" I screamed at them "you fucking what?" he said as dad came at me with a punch, she shouted "go on Ed" I looked at her with utmost hate in my face and said "and you! You evil twisted bitch."

With that dad shouted "don't you dare talk to your mother like that?"

With that I just lost it, and screamed "MOTHER! WHAT! That thing! She is no mother of mine. My mothers worth a million to that tart so don't insult me or my mother."

With that dad grabbed me by the neck, with her screaming "don't let her talk to me like that Ed, he grabbed my neck tighter, dragged me to the door opened it and slung me out.

I cried with the pain of my leg, and the freedom, the light at the end of the tunnel.

In tears I managed to get up, holding the gate, next thing the door opened I froze for a minute, a carrier bag came hurling at me, "that's all your taking now piss off" he shouted.

I started to walk slowly with my leg swollen, and in pain, I just walked anywhere to get away from them, after stopping and starting I got to the local railway station, I sat in the waiting room, I lay my bag on the seat as I clutched it and fell asleep, next thing I woke up it was dark, I just lie down and fell asleep again, exhausted hungry, and scared.

Next I knew it was morning, people looking over me, "are you alright dear?" they asked.

I looked up with a grin, "I'll be better than I have been in a long time now thank you" I said.

And lay down again. I heard people say "oh poor girl look at her do you think she's run away? Or been in a fight? Look at her face bruised and swollen."

As I heard another say look at her leg that's swollen and bruised.

Their voices became a muffled sound as I fell back to sleep.

In time I was woken by the station master, "Hello there love do you know you have been here for few days now, slept the whole time." I sat up "ouch" I said "you've been in the wars it looks like" he said as he handed me a cup of tea, "here drink this down love, a nice hot cup of tea looks like you could do with it" he said.

"Now tell me what your name is and where you are from?" he said.

I looked and said "don't worry mate."

Next thing there was a police man "Hello there" he said "you have caused a bit of a concern sleeping here the station master thought you had moved in" I smiled and said "not quite." "Can we take you home?" he asked then another police man came in too.

I panicked and said "no I'm not going back there." ok calm down" they said "we are to here to help you."

"I'd rather jump under the next train" I said as a figure of speech.

"Oh dear that bad?" they both said.

"Well come down to the station with us and we'll get you a nice hot drink and a nice meal, get your face and leg sorted and we'll go from there, yes?" they both said.

I agreed.

They helped me to the police car.

And off we went to the station.

I was given a hot drink and a meal from the canteen.

They asked what had happened and I told them. They asked what did I want them to do about this, I said nothing now I was only to glad to get away.

They understood and took me to the hospital, I didn't want my leg in plaster or cast, and so they put a tight fit support bandage on it, and gave me some pain killers.

They asked me where I could go and I said "may be my bro's" they asked where he lived and took me.

As we got there they helped me out of the car at Roy's, the policeman knocked, my sister in law Ellie answered. "God what's happened to you?" She said.

"Roy's at work now but he'll be in by 5 or 6 o'clock" she said. "That's ok" said the policeman.

"But she'll be ok with you, yes?"

"Yes sure" Ellie said, they wished me good luck and said "if you needed to talk to telephone the number they gave or call at the station" then went on their way.

Ellie asked what had happened as she put the kettle on as I started to tell her. Ellie was a sweet person, as I was telling her of my ordeal he shouted, "Bastards" she said "I know with a things Roy's told me they need shooting" she said.

She asked About Martin and I explained I hadn't seen him in weeks now, well over a month, as the tears rolled down my face, and Ellie sat and comforted me.

After a while Roy came in looked at me "What the fuck's happened to you had a row with a bus?" He asked.

I told him most and what I have is all they'd give me, regards to clothes, by now the steam was coming out of his ears "stay there he said be back in a minute" next thing he was gone out the door like a bull in a china shop.

On his return he had his mate D.C, "Come on girl get in the car we'll go get your stuff." I looked in horror "come on they won't touch you while we're there the bastards."

Hesitating I went with them.

He pulled up outside I froze.

"I can't face them" I said.

"Come on" said D.C "They touch you I'll knock the pair of them out."

We walked towards the door "your leg? Did they do that?" asked D.C "yes" I said "he did it."

We got to the door, Roy knocked as he did Bumble was looking out of the window.

Dad came to the door "what you lot fucking want?" he asked.

"Her clothes you evil bastard" Roy said and pushed the door open, "go on go get what's yours" Roy and D.C told me. But I froze I started to shake and feel sick, D.C put his arm around me "come on girl I'll come with you" he said as he pushed passed dad.

Helping me up the stairs I shoved all my stuff in a case, and carrier bags I had in the wardrobe, a lot of my stuff was missing but I didn't care I just wanted to get out.

I really couldn't wait to get out of there. This house, this abuse mentally and physically was at an end......I started to feel at ease with Roy and D.C. at my side. Relief I started to cry with relief..... it was all at an end.........

The light at the end of the tunnel...........

Days passed and my leg was swollen, but got better as each day passed, I wanted to get round to Martins but because the time had passed, I was worried about being rejected. I agreed to wait till my leg was much better another week or so, Ellie came with me to the doctors on a few occasions, when I saw one of Martins old school mates.

I asked him had he seen Martin he said "yes you stood him up he's got another girl friend now" I just burst into tears "I never stood him up" I cried "oh well too late now" he said.

Ellie putting her arm around me she said "Don't cry", we will try and sort it out soon, I knew new he was lying and I should not believe him, but I was frightened to find out now as the weeks had gone into months and I was afraid of rejection. I was very fond of Martin but I couldn't cope with all this now, but no matter what people told me. I knew that they were lying. I new Martin better than that, he was too much of a gentleman. And I new my own mind, and what my heart told me. These people were just malicious.

As each day went by I couldn't cope with everything that had happened to me. My relief of being away from dad and Bumble and the horrific life I endured and the grief of loosing Martin. Everything got too much to handle, and I fell to pieces.

Because of dad and Bumble I lost my closest friend my companion, My Martin........

Since I have wrote this book, for the first time in our lives my siblings and I have felt we are all able to talk of the mental and physical Abuse we all endured as children; after so many years of bottling this horrific period of our lives, that has affected us all.

That as we all continued our lives the way we knew how blocking the abuse to carry on. On a day to day basis our history was not part of any day to day conversation, each one afraid to upset the other to recall this period of our lives; some very strong feelings have been felt between us, not knowing how each other really felt until now.

The hurt each of us feel not being allowed to mourn or grieve for our beloved mother. Never being allowed to mention her name or have a photograph of her. This is still as painful today as it was all those years ago; but thankfully we can all recall the love and happiness our mum showed us, it was the love she gave that none of us ever forgot.

That helped us to survive the life we endured, as time went and we found each other we became a very close family.

One of my siblings feels very strong to air his views on how he feels today, in which he states; I would like to say that the only good thing my dad had done, was to be a sperm donor to the most wonderful, caring thoughtful brothers and sisters that trod this earth.

Whom I love, with the utmost respect; their partners also, have been there for me twenty four seven, no if's, no butt's, they are there whatever.

I honestly cannot thank all you enough for being my family.

God Bless You All

Before I die I would also like to sayif I ever found dads grave I would have my favourite tipple [brandy] in my right hand, I would pour half the bottle on his grave with the left hand, and I would urinate on his Head Stone....

Love Roy

I think the words of Roy sums up to how he feels about our father....

www.ingramcontent.com/pod-product-compliance
Lightning Source LLC
Chambersburg PA
CBHW061244280526
45784CB00002B/627